The Jossey-Bass/AHA Press Series translates the latest ideas on health care management into practical and actionable terms. Together, Jossey-Bass and the American Hospital Association offer these essential resources for the health care leaders of today and tomorrow.

# Privacy and Confidentiality of Health Information

# Privacy and Confidentiality of Health Information

JILL CALLAHAN DENNIS

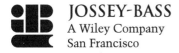

JOSSEY-BASS
A Wiley Company
San Francisco

press

Library of Congress Cataloging-in-Publication Data
Dennis, Jill Callahan.
    Privacy and confidentiality of health information / Jill Callahan Dennis.
      p. cm.
    Includes bibliographical references and index.
    ISBN 0-7879-5278-8 (alk. paper)
    1. Medical records—Access control. 2. Privacy, Right of. 3. Confidential communications—Access control. I. Title.
    R864 .D45 2000
    174'.2—dc21
                                                                        00-009556

*HB Printing*    10 9 8 7 6 5 4 3 2 1                    FIRST EDITION

The Jossey-Bass Health Series

# CONTENTS

Preface    xi

The Author    xv

1 Introduction: Why Privacy and Confidentiality Matter    1

2 The Legal Underpinnings    9

3 Navigating the Confidentiality Minefield    25

4 Developing Confidentiality Policies and Procedures    35

5 Confidentiality Training    67

6 The Future    77

Appendix    81

Notes    97

References    99

Index    101

In my work as a consultant, I've had the honor of seeing, first-hand, the commitment of countless health care providers, health information managers, and risk managers who respect their patients' privacy and work to improve systems for protecting the confidentiality of patients' health information. This book is dedicated to those heroes, who turn confidentiality theory into reality every day.

# PREFACE

As we enter a new millennium, we face fundamentally important questions about how our increasingly information-driven society will impact our individual freedoms. Will the faster and freer flow of information made possible by new technologies only make life better? Or will the price—paid in the loss of privacy—be too high?

Already, uses of our health information are expanding beyond the original purposes for which the information was collected. Witness the growth of database marketing to sell certain medical products or pharmaceuticals to classes of patients with a particular disease. Information technology's application to what were previously paper-based medical records has made it possible to do far more with that information. This has tremendous benefits in supporting research and quality improvement, and has resulted in administrative efficiencies as well as improvements in provider-to-provider communication. But these same technologies present potential risks to patient confidentiality by making it easier to share information inappropriately.

This book is designed to explore emerging risks to confidentiality and privacy. It describes potential solutions to the most common risks, and summarizes some of the existing resources to help you avoid breaches on confidentiality—whether you work in acute care, long-term care, ambulatory care, or home care settings.

*Chapter One* sets the stage by examining how public concern for privacy is growing and why every health care organization must be demonstrably concerned with protecting patient or client confidentiality.

*Chapter Two* describes the underlying laws, regulations, ethical codes, and case law that form a legal framework for our information-handling and dissemination practices.

*Chapter Three* discusses common breaches of confidentiality, why they occur, and how you can determine the extent to which your own organization is at risk of breaching confidentiality.

*Chapter Four* offers guidelines for developing appropriate policies and procedures to prevent the confidentiality breach, examined both from the standpoint of various types of information users and various information and communication technologies, such as computer-based patient records, wireless communication devices, e-mail systems, and more.

*Chapter Five* examines the need to train employees and the medical staff to protect the information they generate and handle. The importance of top-down commitment to confidentiality is discussed, as is the need to provide confidentiality training to volunteers and vendors who handle your patients' information.

*Chapter Six* addresses a few of the most interesting emerging issues and technologies, and discusses the near-future forecast for legislation and regulation.

Finally, an *Appendix* offers a compendium of resources that can improve your organization's ability to protect patients' confidentiality: a sample protocol for conducting an internal risk assessment of your health information systems, print materials, videos, computer-based training, association resources, and Internet-based resources. New tools are being developed constantly that can assist your staff in better protecting patient information. The Appendix offers a head start in locating the resources you need.

Although the protection of patient confidentiality has always been profoundly important to every health care organization, the recently issued federal Privacy Rule is driving a renewed (and mandated) interest in examining internal systems for protecting patient information. This book is designed to help us close the gaps, strengthen the weaknesses, educate our staffs, and better meet our obligations to patients—who trust us not only with their health, but also with their most private information.

## ACKNOWLEDGMENTS

Writing is part pleasure and part agony but mostly long, hard work, complicated by a changing regulatory scene. Several people made this project possible. Thanks to Andy Pasternack and the staff of Jossey-Bass Publishers, and Rick Hill of American Hospital Publishing for their enthusiasm, patience, and expert assistance. Day-to-day encouragement and support came from my parents Seaber and Hazel Callahan, my client and friend Mary Ryan of Reliance National Insurance Company, my husband Ron Dennis, the reviewers, and especially my friend and partner Bud Marker. Thanks are also owed to the communications staff at the American Health Information Management Association (AHIMA) for enabling me to "think on paper" about confidentiality in past issues of *In Confidence* and the *Journal of AHIMA*.

*Parker, Colorado*                                   Jill Callahan Dennis
*July 2000*

# THE AUTHOR

Jill Callahan Dennis is a principal of Health Risk Advantage in Parker, Colorado and serves as chair of the legislative committee of the American Health Information Management Association and the Confidentiality Toolkit Task Force of the American Society for Health Risk Management. She is a contributing author to *Health Information: Management of a Strategic Resource* (1996) and the principal author of the CD-ROM *Managing Risks in Clinical Documentation and Health Information* (1996).

# Privacy and Confidentiality of Health Information

# Introduction: Why Privacy and Confidentiality Matter

I f it seems to you that the world has gotten smaller in recent years, you are in good company. Advances in computer technology and telecommunications have made it as easy to communicate with a professional colleague halfway around the world as it is to make a local phone call.

## IS PRIVACY A REASONABLE EXPECTATION?

With just a few strokes on a keyboard, we can access information on an infinite variety of subjects—and people. Often, the information is not adequately protected from misuse. In fact, our laws have not kept pace with today's information-rich environment. In many cases, we often haven't even defined "misuse."

At the same time, patients are becoming more sensitive to the uses and handling of their health information. In 1995, members of Harvard Community Health Plan were angered to learn that physicians at the health plan routinely put detailed psychiatric counseling notes into computerized medical records that were accessible to many of the health maintenance organization's (HMO's) employees—not just the members' therapists (Bass, 1995).[1]

Even though the public is, for the most, only vaguely aware of the many uses to which their health information is put, their concerns for confidentiality are growing. Those concerns result in increasing media attention to confidentiality and increased interest in the subject by lawmakers.

It may well be positive that public interest in confidentiality encourages all of us to be more knowledgeable about our health information and how it is used. However, the day-to-day responsibility for protecting patient confidentiality can be left neither to the public nor to Congress. That responsibility must fall squarely on the shoulders of every health care provider. We must identify potential and actual abuses, strengthen our information systems, and minimize the risks of confidentiality breaches.

Consumers are often unaware of the uses to which their health information is put. Even health care providers sometimes don't appreciate all of the ways in which their own health information can be used. Consider this case reported by Givens (1997) from the files of the San Diego–based Privacy Rights Clearinghouse: "A physician in private practice was puzzled about why she had trouble getting insurance for her office. Then she found out she'd been wrongly coded in a national medical database as suffering from Alzheimer's disease, and with a history of heart disease."

Most patients have some vague understanding that their information is sent to their health insurer as justification for payment. However, most are unaware that the information provided to certain insurers may be passed along, once again, to the Medical Information Bureau (MIB). The MIB is a collective database made up of coded medical information supplied by participating insurers. Because this database is used by participating companies as an underwriting tool (that is, in making decisions about insurability), the information can come back to haunt unsuspecting patients—whether that information is correct or incorrect. See Figure 1.1 for more information on the Medical Information Bureau.

## CONSUMER EXPECTATIONS

Consumers' concerns over the use of health information for wide-ranging purposes—many unrelated to the provision of actual care—have been growing in recent years, along with consumer fears over the general erosion

**Figure 1.1. How Patients Can Find Out Whether the Medical Information Bureau Has Information About Them.**

Patients can find out whether the Medical Information Bureau has information about them by contacting

In the United States:
**Medical Information Bureau**
PO Box 105, Essex Station
Boston, MA 02112
617–426–3660

In Canada:
**Medical Information Bureau**
330 University Avenue
Toronto, Ontario
Canada M5G 1R7
416–597–0590

of privacy. A 1993 Louis Harris poll, commissioned by Equifax (Equifax, 1993), reported that 79 percent of the American public is worried about their privacy. Forty-nine percent of the participants reported that they were "very" worried, and an additional thirty-nine percent described themselves as "somewhat" worried about the threat to personal privacy.

Government agencies have begun to respond to those concerns. A Task Force on Privacy was established in 1990 by the assistant secretary for Planning and Evaluation, Department of Health and Human Services, to report on the privacy of private sector health records. Another DHHS group established in the early 1990s, the Workgroup on Electronic Data Interchange (WEDI), was formed to address the need to protect medical claims being submitted electronically.

President Clinton's 1993 Health Care Reform Task Forces also considered the need to protect health information. Numerous legislative proposals since then have called for greater protections for health information.

And in 1996, the Health Insurance Portability and Accountability Act set the stage for the recently issued proposed rule setting standards for the security of individual health information and electronic signature use by health plans and health care providers (USDHHS, 1998), as well as the proposed rule on privacy of health information (USDHHS, 1999).

## OPERATIONAL DIFFICULTIES IN PROTECTING CONFIDENTIALITY

Clearly, public attention to the confidentiality and privacy of health information is at an all-time high. But although most would agree that private health information should be handled appropriately, there is much disagreement over what that really means. For example, when families gather at a hospital where an elderly parent has been admitted, it is common for the adult children to assume that they should have automatic access to any and all health information about their parent. However, if that parent is competent, he or she should be deciding what information, if any, is shared with the children.

If a drug manufacturer mails patients literature about a drug the manufacturer knows they are taking, based on a pharmacy's database, is that misuse? Or is it a public service? Would patients answer differently depending on whether their drug was for heart disease or AIDS? Would patients be surprised that their prescription information was being used for marketing purposes, or would they think it a perfectly logical and appropriate activity?

Expectations aside, there are operational difficulties in protecting the confidentiality of health information. One difficulty arises from the sheer number of people with access to health information. Dozens of health care workers have access to the typical hospitalized patient's health information. On a nursing unit, all nursing staff may have ready access to the information of all unit patients, whether or not they are caring for that patient. In a medical practice, all employees of the practice might have potential access to the information.

Often, not all those who have potential access actually need that information. Unless an employee is involved in caring for a particular patient or in processing their health information (for example, for billing, transcription, or other business purposes), that employee should ordinarily not have access to the patient's record. But particularly in a manual, paper-based record-keeping system, it may be impractical to segregate records physically in a way that prevents unauthorized staff from having access.

Even in computerized health information systems, the system's design sometimes does not bar unauthorized staff from accessing a particular patient's information. For example, unless the system has a way of recording who is "officially" involved in caring for the patient, it may be possible for any physician, nurse, laboratory technician, or other health care professional to look up any patient's information—even patients for whom that professional is not providing care.

Yet another operational difficulty in maintaining patient confidentiality is the challenge of educating health care staff about their role in protecting patients' privacy and confidentiality. The orientation sessions we offer new employees have become so overstuffed with information mandated by accrediting and regulatory agencies that it's difficult to find the time to discuss confidentiality in anything more than the most rudimentary fashion. Unfortunately, often that orientation is both the *first* *and last* time an employee hears about patient confidentiality. Chapter Five discusses the importance of this training, and includes recommendations for content.

## The Impact of Information Technology on Confidentiality

The growth of computerized health information systems brings a new urgency to the need to assure patient confidentiality. One of the benefits of computerizing that information—easier and more rapid access—also poses a potential threat to confidentiality. In a manual record-keeping environment, the labor involved in retrieving information from paper records served as a deterrent of sorts. To gather information on a group of patients would require manually retrieving the records, poring through the data, and recording or copying what was needed. In an electronic system without carefully designed access and audit controls, retrieving data on a group of patients may be accomplished almost instantaneously and invisibly.

Few would argue that the risks of computerization outweigh the benefits. Still, careful thought must be given to the design of safeguards for computerized patient data so that these systems enhance rather than detract from the security and confidentiality of health information. The proposed security standards published by the Department of Health and Human Services (USDHHS, 1998) will set baseline standards for those safeguards.

## The Impact of Other Forces

The growth of information technology is not the only force affecting societal concern for privacy and confidentiality in health care. The growth of integrated delivery systems, in which previously independent health care providers and facilities are grouped under a single corporate umbrella, has resulted in certain health information being compiled in corporate databases for management purposes. For example, some integrated delivery systems collect data on unusual occurrences or incidents at their member facilities for use in detecting patterns and trends that may indicate the need for new procedures, policies, or staff training. Patients are rarely aware that the details of their treatment could end up in a "home office" database across the country from where they received their treatment.

The deepening penetration of managed care into the health insurance marketplace has also created new demands for information. Now instead of merely receiving a coded bill for services already provided, utilization management staff at the managed care organization are contacting the health care provider while treatment is under way, requesting information to justify that treatment, and, in many cases, influencing the actual treatment provided. How much information is enough to justify payment of the bill? This is a problem many health care case managers are struggling with as they attempt to protect the patient's privacy while avoiding a payment denial.

Privacy and Confidentiality of Health Information

## The Implications of a Confidentiality Breach

Just why should we be so concerned about confidentiality? Don't patients expect to yield some of their privacy whenever they seek treatment? Probably so—to the extent that information is needed to pay the bills. But patients can also be harmed by careless or inappropriate disclosures of health information:

- A Maryland banker was accused of cross-referencing a list of cancer patients against a list of outstanding loans at his bank—and then calling in the loans (Givens, 1997).

- A staff physician at a New Jersey hospital was stigmatized when his HIV status was discussed by hospital personnel (*Estate of Behringer* v. *Princeton Medical Center,* 1991).

- A number of political candidates over the years have been publicly embarrassed by the unauthorized release of their health histories; most recently Rep. Nydia Velasquez (Democrat–New York), whose records of a past hospitalization for attempted suicide were faxed to the media during her campaign.

Gathering statistics about the harm caused to patients by breaches of confidentiality is complicated by the fact that the patient may not know how, or from where, the disclosure originated. They may also be reluctant to complain about such breaches because of a desire to avoid compounding the embarrassment or harm by perpetuating the discussion. And most health care facilities are not likely to admit voluntarily to a breach of confidentiality that has not yet been discovered by either the patient or the public at large.

Regardless of whether patients are aware of these breaches, they do exist. Twenty-four percent of the health leaders participating in the 1993 Harris/Equifax survey mentioned earlier claimed to be "aware of violations of the confidentiality of individuals' medical records from inside an organization that embarrassed or harmed the individual" (Equifax, 1993).

Patients are not the only ones potentially harmed by a confidentiality or security breach. Health care providers who have been shown to be responsible for such breaches, through the actions of their employees, have been successfully sued and subjected to administrative sanctions. Some of these cases are discussed in Chapter Three.

Jury awards and monetary penalties aside, most health care providers recognize that maintaining their patients' confidentiality is a matter of trust and an important factor in maintaining a positive public reputation. We all stand to gain by implementing practices and policies that protect health information from inappropriate uses. Helping you accomplish that in your organization is the purpose of this book.

# The Legal Underpinnings

Intuitively, affording patients privacy and handling their information with respect seems appropriate. But there are laws, regulations, ethical codes, and even case law that, taken together, impose actual legally recognized duties upon health care providers to maintain confidentiality and privacy.

Although at the time of this writing there is not yet a comprehensive, uniform federal law protecting the confidentiality of all health care information (although several bills in Congress would establish federal law on the subject, and recently proposed federal rules would protect part of that information), a number of state laws address the subject, as do Medicare's conditions of participation and accrediting agency standards. In addition, federal regulations tightly control the disclosure of information about treatment given in alcohol and drug abuse programs.

Accreditation standards also require that health information be kept confidential. For example, the Joint Commission on Accreditation of Healthcare Organizations (JCAHO) requires health care organizations to have a "functioning mechanism designed to safeguard records and information against loss, destruction, tampering, and unauthorized access or use" (Joint Commission on Accreditation of Healthcare Organizations [JCAHO], 1995).

Ethical standards also address the health care provider's duty to handle health information with care. Physicians, for example, are required by the Hippocratic oath to maintain confidentiality.[2] The American Hospital

Association's (AHA) Patient's Bill of Rights addresses the health facility's obligation.[3] The American Health Information Management Association's Code of Ethics sets the standard for health information management (HIM) professionals.[4]

To understand fully the obligation to keep the patient's health information confidential, we need to understand just exactly what information *is* and *is not* confidential. Simply putting information within a health record does not make that information confidential. After all, some of the information that ends up in the patient's record is not even health- or treatment-related. The date of a patient's clinic visit would not necessarily be confidential, nor would his address or date of birth. (Even though these may not be "legally" confidential, there may be situations in which a provider would still appropriately decline to respond to requests for this information. For example, in the past many hospitals automatically published notices of birth in the local newspaper, listing the parents' name and address and the sex or name of the child. These days, perhaps because infant abductions have captured public attention, fewer hospitals do this, even with the consent of the parents.)

Unfortunately, determining what is and what is not confidential is not always as simple as it might seem. And the rules may vary with the treatment setting. For example, for substance-abuse treatment facilities, the very fact of a patient's admission for treatment is confidential, according to federal regulations, and may not be disclosed without patient authorization except under very limited circumstances.[5] But generally, informational items unrelated to the treatment provided, such as the patient's name, address, next of kin, or other guarantor information, are not considered confidential. This would hold true under the recently published proposed rules on security and electronic signatures, as well as the November 2, 1999 *Federal Register*'s proposed rule on privacy of individually identifiable health information. The proposed definition of *health information* used in those proposed rules can be found in Figure 2.1.

Health information is not the only confidential information in our organizations. Incident or occurrence reports and the resulting investiga-

**Figure 2.1. Definition of Health Information from Health Care Financing Administration's Proposed Rules.**

The Health Care Financing Administration's proposed rules on security and electronic signature standards define health information as "any information, whether oral or recorded in any form or medium, that

1. Is created or received by a health care provider, health plan, public health authority, employer, life insurer, school or university, or health care clearinghouse; and

2. Relates to the past, present, or future physical or mental health or condition of an individual, the provision of health care to an individual, or the past, present, or future payment for the provision of health care to an individual."

*Source: Federal Register,* August 12, 1998, volume 63, number 155, p. 43264.

tions are kept confidential to the extent permitted by state law so that we can learn from mistakes and address systemic weaknesses, and so staff members will not be discouraged from reporting such occurrences. And as McCann (1993) observes, peer review and quality improvement-related records, such as those found in some committee and task force minutes and credentialing files, also must be kept confidential to encourage candor in monitoring, managing, and improving the quality of care.

## SOME IMPORTANT FEDERAL LAWS AND REGULATIONS ON CONFIDENTIALITY

In developing our organization's policies and procedures to protect confidential information, we must ensure that those policies adhere to current federal and state laws and regulations on the subject. The most important federal laws and regulations are summarized as follows.

*Freedom of Information Act.* The Freedom of Information Act (FOIA) requires that records of the executive branch of the federal government be available to the public, except for matters falling within nine explicitly exempted areas in the act. Under certain circumstances, medical records may be exempt from FOIA requirements. One of the exempt categories includes "personnel and medical files and similar files, the disclosure of which would constitute a clearly unwarranted invasion of personal privacy" (Freedom of Information Act, 1977). To qualify as an "unwarranted invasion of personal privacy" (1) the information must be contained in a personnel, medical, or similar file; (2) disclosure of the information must constitute an invasion of personal privacy; and (3) the severity of the invasion must outweigh the public's interest in disclosure. Interpreting this test has been the subject of litigation.[6]

*Privacy Act of 1974.* The Privacy Act was designed to give U.S. citizens some control over the information collected about them by the federal government. It permits individuals to find out what information about them has been collected, see and have a copy of that information, correct or amend the information, and exercise limited control of the disclosure of that information to other parties.[7] Health care organizations operated by the federal government are bound by the act, including Department of Defense health care facilities, Veterans' Administration health facilities, and Indian Health Service facilities. It also applies to record systems that are operated under contract to a federal government agency; for example, a disease registry operated under a grant from the Department of Health and Human Services.

*Regulations on Confidentiality of Alcohol and Drug Abuse Records.* These regulations, restricting disclosures of patient health information without patient authorization, apply to facilities that provide alcohol or drug abuse diagnosis, treatment, or referral for treatment. For a health care organization to fall under this definition, it must offer either (1) an identified unit that provides alcohol or drug abuse diagnosis, treatment, or referral for treatment, or (2) medical personnel or other staff whose primary function is the provision of alcohol or drug abuse diagnosis, treatment, or referral for treatment and who are identified as such providers. General hospitals and clinics are not considered to fall under this definition unless they have either an identified unit for this type of diagnosis or treatment, or providers whose primary function is the provision of those types of services.

The regulations apply to health information obtained by "federally assisted programs," but because the definition of this includes all Medicare-certified facilities or organizations receiving funds provided by any federal department or agency, the regulations apply to almost all substance-abuse programs that meet the other requirements of the definition.

These regulations prohibit the disclosure of substance-abuse patient information unless permitted by the regulations or authorized by the patient. The regulations also dictate the specific content for valid authorizations to release health information. To be valid, the authorization must include

- The specific name or general designation of the program or person permitted to make the disclosure.
- The name or title of the individual or the name of the organization to which disclosure is to be made.
- The name of the patient.
- The purpose of the disclosure.
- How much and what kind of information is to be disclosed.
- The signature of the patient and, when required for a patient who is a minor,[8] the signature of a person authorized to give consent under §2.14 of the regulations; or, when required for a patient who is incompetent or deceased, the signature of a person authorized to sign under §2.15 in lieu of the patient.
- The date on which the consent (authorization) is signed.
- A statement that the consent is subject to revocation at any time, except to the extent that the program or person which is to make the disclosure has already acted in reliance on it. Acting in reliance includes the provision of treatment services in reliance on a valid consent to disclose information to a third party payer.
- The date, event, or condition upon which the consent will expire if not revoked before. This date, event, or condition must ensure that the consent will last no longer than reasonably necessary to serve the purpose for which it is given.[9]

After this list was published, many health care organizations adopted these elements as the content of their general authorization for release of health information, applying to all releases of health information, rather than use separate forms for separate purposes. This eliminated the need to have special authorizations for special purposes.

Each disclosure must be accompanied by a notice specified in the regulations on confidentiality of alcohol and drug abuse records. That notice prohibits redisclosure. It instructs the information recipients that they may not redisclose the information to anyone else or use the information for anything but its intended purpose, because the records are protected by the federal rules. The notice states: "This information has been disclosed to you from records whose confidentiality is protected by Federal law. Federal regulations (42 CFR Part 2) prohibit you from making any further disclosure of it without the specific written consent of the person to whom it pertains, or as otherwise permitted by such regulations. A general authorization for the release of medical or other information is *not* sufficient for this purpose."

As mentioned earlier, there are some exceptions to the general prohibition against disclosure. For example, the regulations allow disclosure to medical personnel to treat a condition that "poses an immediate threat to the health of the patient" (see §2.51 of the regulations mentioned in the previous paragraph). Records of these disclosures must be maintained and must include the patient's name or case number, date and time of disclosure, description of circumstances requiring emergency disclosure, description of information disclosed, the identity of the party receiving the information, and the identity of the party disclosing the information (§2.51[e]). There are also some provisions for interagency disclosures (for example, to the Food and Drug Administration), research, and Medicare or Medicaid audits (§2.51–2.53).

*Health Insurance Portability and Accountability Act (HIPAA).* In 1996, Congress passed the act commonly referred to as HIPAA (Public Law 104–191). As part of that act, Congress added a new section to Title XI of the Social Security Act, entitled "Administrative Simplification." The purpose of the Administrative Simplification amendment was to improve the efficiency and effectiveness of the health care system by stimulating the development of standards to facilitate electronic maintenance and transmission of health information. The act directs the secretary of the Department of Health and Human Services to adopt standards for electronically

Privacy and Confidentiality of Health Information

maintained health information, as well as standards for electronic signatures, and other matters such as unique health identifiers and code sets.

As an outgrowth of HIPAA, the secretary formulated a five-part strategy for developing and implementing these standards.

Step one involved establishing interdepartmental teams to identify existing standards and evaluate them for potential adoption. The teams consulted with various industry associations and groups.

In step two, the teams developed recommendations for the standards to be adopted.

In step three, the proposed rules were published in the *Federal Register,* with a sixty-day comment period. The proposed rules on security and electronic signatures were published August 12, 1998. And because Congress failed to enact federal confidentiality legislation by the deadline imposed by HIPAA, a proposed rule on privacy of individually identifiable health information was published November 3, 1999.

In step four, DHHS will analyze public comments and publish the final rules in the *Federal Register.*

In the final step, step five, the standards will be distributed and implementation guides will be prepared and distributed. As this book goes to press, we are currently in step four—awaiting the publication of the final rules.

## PROPOSED RULES ON SECURITY AND PRIVACY

The proposed rules on security and on privacy are as follows. It is difficult to predict just how closely the final rules will follow what has been proposed, but it is likely that the major categories that describe essential security features will not change in any major way.

*Proposed Rule: Security and Electronic Signature Standards.* Pursuant to the requirements of HIPAA, on August 12, 1998, the secretary of the Department of Health and Human Services published the proposed standards for electronically maintained health information (as well as proposed standards for electronic signatures). The regulations, once finalized, will apply to health care providers, health plans, and health care (data) clearinghouses. At this point, it appears that publication of the final rule will occur in mid- to late 2000, after all comments on the proposed rule are analyzed.

Certain procedures, safeguards, and technical security services will be required under these regulations. Tables from the August 12 Notice of Proposed Rules which summarize the proposed security-related proposed and methods of implementation appear in Figures 2.2 through 2.4.

The regulations are expected to apply to all electronically-maintained health information in health care organizations.

In reviewing Figures 2.2 through 2.4, many readers will discover that they already have some of these required elements in place, but it is likely

**Figure 2.2.  Administrative Procedures to Guard Data Integrity, Confidentiality, and Availability.**

| | |
|---|---|
| Certification | |
| Chain of trust partner agreement | |
| Contingency plan (all listed implementation features must be implemented) | Applications and data criticality analysis. Data backup plan. Disaster recovery plan. Emergency mode operation plan. Testing and revision. |
| Formal mechanism for processing records | |
| Information access control (all listed features must be implemented) | Access authorization. Access establishment. Access modification. |
| Internal audit | |
| Personnel security (all listed features must be implemented) | Supervision of maintenance personnel by authorized, knowledgeable person. Maintenance of record of access authorizations. |

Privacy and Confidentiality of Health Information

|  | Proper access authorization of operating and, in some cases, maintenance personnel. Personnel clearance procedure. Personnel security policy and procedure. System users, including maintenance personnel, trained in security. |
| --- | --- |
| Security configuration management (all listed features must be implemented) | Documentation. Hardware and software installation and maintenance review and testing for security features. Inventory. Security testing. Virus checking. |
| Security incident procedures (all listed features must be implemented) | Report procedures. Response procedures. |
| Security management process (all listed features must be implemented) | Risk analysis. Risk management. Sanction policy. Security policy. |
| Termination procedures (all listed features must be implemented) | Combination locks changed. Removal from access lists. Removal of user account(s). Turn in of keys, token, or cards that allow access. |
| Training (all listed features must be implemented) | Awareness training for all personnel (including management). Periodic security reminders. User education concerning virus protection. User education in importance of monitoring log-in success and failure, and how to report discrepancies. User education in password management. |

## Figure 2.3. Physical Safeguards to Guard Data Integrity, Confidentiality, and Availability.

| Requirement | Implementation |
|---|---|
| Assigned security responsibility | |
| Media controls (all listed implementation features must be implemented) | Access control. Accountability (tracking mechanism). Data backup. Data storage. Disposal. |
| Physical access controls (limited access) (all listed features must be implemented) | Disaster recovery. Emergency mode operation. Equipment control (into and out of site). Facility security plan. Procedures for verifying access authorizations prior to physical access. Maintenance records. Need-to-know procedures for personnel access. Sign-in for visitors and escort, if appropriate. Testing and revision. |
| Policy or guideline on work station use | |
| Secure work station location | |
| Security awareness training | |

**Figure 2.4.  Technical Security Services and Mechanisms.**

| Requirement | Implementation |
|---|---|
| Access control (The following implementation feature must be implemented: procedure for emergency access. In addition, at least one of the following three implementation features must be implemented: context-based access, role-based access, user-based access. The use of encryption is optional.) | Context-based access. Encryption. Procedure for emergency access. Role-based access. User-based access. |
| Audit controls | |
| Authorization control (At least one of the listed implementation features must be implemented.) | Role-based access. User-based access. |
| Data authentication | |
| Entity authentication (The following implementation features must be implemented: automatic log-off, unique user identification. In addition, at least one of the other listed implementation features must be implemented.) | Automatic log-off. Biometric. Password. PIN. Telephone call-back. Token. Unique user identification. |
| Communications/network controls (The following implementation features must be implemented: integrity controls, message authentication. If communications or networking is employed, one of the following implementation features must be implemented: access controls, encryption. In addition, if using a network, the following four implementation features must be implemented: alarm, audit trail, entity authentication, event reporting.) | Access controls. Alarm. Audit trail. Encryption. Entity authentication. Event reporting. Integrity controls. Message authentication. |

that better documentation of security procedures and better (and more comprehensive) training in information security and confidentiality will be necessary.

*Proposed Rule: Standards for Privacy of Individually Identifiable Health Information.* Under HIPAA, the Department of Health and Human Services was given the authority and responsibility to promulgate rules governing the privacy of health information if Congress failed to pass a privacy statute within three years of HIPAA's enactment. That deadline passed without successful legislation on August 21, 1999. As a result, the secretary of the Department of Health and Human Services issued a proposed rule on November 3, 1999.

The proposed rule's provisions apply to health plans, health care clearinghouses, and any health care provider who transmits health information in electronic form, but the provisions cover only individually identifiable health information that is (or has been) maintained or transmitted in electronic form. Unfortunately, this creates a situation in which only part of the health information in a single patient's medical record may be protected—the part that is (or has been) electronically maintained or transmitted. Many groups commenting on the proposed rule (such as the American Health Information Management Association) have called for the rule's coverage to be expanded to *all* individually identifiable health information of these covered entities, but the final rule has not yet been issued.

The proposed rule seeks to define and limit the circumstances in which an individual's health information may be used or disclosed. At the same time, the rule relaxes the preexisting requirements associated with certain administrative and financial uses of the health information—such as the use of health information to obtain payment for health care services, and the use of the information for internal quality improvement purposes.

The proposed rule also seeks to give patients an organized process for obtaining a copy of their health information and limits many of the internal and external disclosures by imposing a *"minimum necessary"* standard. With some exceptions, the permitted uses and disclosures of health information would be limited to the minimum amount of information necessary to achieve the purpose for which the information is being requested. This standard, likely to be incorporated into the final rule, will require health care providers to tighten their procedures for information disclosure and to use good judgment in fulfilling requests for information. This will result in a need for more and better training of the staff members involved in disclosing information, and will require health care information systems staff and vendors to design tighter access control measures into their computer systems. For example, it will no longer be acceptable for most health care employees to have unlimited and unfettered access to the entire set of health information for any given patient. Access will need to be restricted to information that is necessary for them to do their jobs.

A number of responsibilities are imposed on health care providers and health plans by the proposed rule. Providers and plans must develop a notice of information practices to help educate patients about the entities' information-handling procedures. They must also develop procedures to allow patients to inspect and copy their health information. They must have a mechanism to document all disclosures for purposes other than treatment, payment, and health care operations. There must be a mechanism to permit patients to request amendments or corrections to their health information.

Health care providers and plans will also have to designate a privacy officer who will oversee the organization's compliance with the rules. Certain administrative, technical, and physical safeguards will be required (as outlined in the information security proposed standards), as will internal penalties or sanctions for employee violation of the rules or procedures.

The proposed rule is rather controversial and has drawn over 150,000 industry and public comments. A final rule, reflecting that input, is likely to be made in late-2000.

Will this rule be the final word on the confidentiality of health information? Probably not. The rule may still be superseded if Congress chooses to enact law on this subject. And even if Congress never passes confidentiality legislation, this rule does not preempt more restrictive (that is, stronger) state laws or federal regulations on the subject. The proposed rule therefore acts as a "floor" for, but not a "ceiling" on, privacy protection for health information.

Until we have a more comprehensive federal law covering general health care information, state laws and the final HIPAA rules will probably be our most important resources in developing policies and procedures for preserving confidentiality when dealing with issues other than federally regulated alcohol and drug abuse health information.

## CASE LAW ON CONFIDENTIALITY AND PRIVACY

Case law can be instructive in interpreting existing laws on confidentiality and privacy. The difficulty with case law is that what sets precedent for one jurisdiction does not necessarily apply in any other jurisdiction. However, courts do look to past case law (but are not necessarily bound by results from outside their jurisdictional area) in making their own decisions about cases alleging a breach of confidentiality or invasion of privacy. Some of the most-often quoted cases involving confidentiality and privacy are as follows.

*Estate of Behringer* v. *Princeton Medical Center, 249 N.J. Super. 597, 592 A.2d 1251 (1991).* Behringer, a surgeon at Princeton Medical Center, was diagnosed with AIDS. Behringer's medical record, which included several references to the diagnosis, was kept at the nursing unit with no special protection to prevent browsing by employees. Soon his condition was widely known in the medical center. Behringer sued Princeton Medical Center for its failure to take reasonable steps to protect his confidentiality.

In another case involving a physician harmed by a confidentiality breach, a federal jury in Atlanta recently sided with the physician-patient in a suit alleging breach of confidentiality by his alcoholism-treatment provider (Rankin, 1998). The patient, a Texas physician, was being treated at a Georgia recovery center, a provider specializing in addiction recovery for health care professionals. The physician signed forms authorizing release of certain information to the Texas State Board of Medicine; however, facility staff released certain information compiled *after* the authorization was signed—in other words, they used the authorization prospectively. The defendant argued at trial that because the signed authorization didn't expire until one year after signing, that meant that it authorized the release of all information gathered during that year after signing. Experts for the plaintiff argued that although the authorization could be presented up to one year after signing, it only covered information gathered before or at the time that the authorization was signed. The jury agreed and awarded the physician two hundred thousand dollars in damages.

*Velasquez v. St. Clare's Hospital (Kings County Supreme Court, New York, 1994).* Velasquez was admitted to St. Clare's Hospital in 1991. In 1992, while she was running for election to U.S. House of Representatives, copies of her medical records were distributed to the press, and the facts involving her care, including psychiatric information, were reported by the media. Velasquez sued the hospital for breach of contractual and fiduciary duties of confidentiality, wrongful disclosure, and negligence in failing to maintain the security of her information.

*O'Connor v. Rutland Medical Center (Vermont, 1994).* O'Connor claimed that at least twice, hospital employees discussed her condition, without her consent, with her husband and ex-husband.

*Doe v. Methodist Hospital (Hancock County Superior Court, Indiana, 1992).* According to the complaint, the patient disclosed his positive HIV status to paramedics when he was taken to the hospital after a heart attack. The paramedics noted this on their trip report, which became part of Doe's medical record. Hospital employees reportedly revealed Doe's HIV status to his coworkers, and Doe sued the hospital and some of its employees for invasion of privacy and other wrongful conduct.

Juries and judges use various guides in determining the outcomes of cases. Certainly, laws and regulations, other cases, experts' opinions, the credibility of witnesses, and available facts all factor into their decisions. Other sources that can be used in determining the standard of case law that is applied in judging breach of confidentiality lawsuits are the standards and guidelines published by professional associations. For example, in the Atlanta case just described (Rankin, 1998), guidelines published by the American Health Information Management Association were used as a trial exhibit. Some of the standards and guidelines on confidentiality published by various professional and medical associations are described in the Appendix under the heading "Resources." These should be used by health care providers in developing their own information-handling policies and procedures.

# Navigating the Confidentiality Minefield

Buried beneath the forest of laws, regulations, and professional standards is a minefield of potential disasters. These requirements impose duties on health care providers to manage information in certain ways: to control access, limit disclosure, and handle the information by using prescribed methods. Complicating our compliance with these laws, regulations, and standards is the rapid development of new information technologies—including, of course, the computer.

Confidential information has always been subject to misuse. Holding careless conversations, leaving paper records available where others can see them, failing to secure filed records—all of these were potential problems in the past. Add to this the ability to pull up hundreds of records on a computer monitor in the time it would take to retrieve a single paper record from the Health Information Management Department and the ability to print that information in remote locations, and the potential for damage becomes greater.

Computerizing health care information doesn't necessarily sacrifice confidentiality. Many experts believe that computerization offers the ability to institute access controls more effectively, so only *authorized* parties can view, print, or use that information. The effective deployment of access controls has, however, been problematic for many health care organizations.

Brandt (1996) points out that access to computerized patient information should be permitted according to the "least privilege" principle: users should be granted access only to the specific information and functions they require to do their jobs. And while this makes perfect sense, and in fact is likely to be mandated by the final privacy rules being issued in 2000 by the Department of Health and Human Services, it can be difficult to implement in a fast-paced health care organization where the professionals involved in caring for a single patient may change rapidly as consultations are requested, coverage arrangements take effect after hours, and patient assignments are changed.

## TYPICAL CONFIDENTIALITY, PRIVACY PROBLEMS

Technology has indeed posed some new confidentiality risks. But the most common confidentiality and privacy-related problems have their roots in human behavior.

### Careless Conversations in the Workplace

Unfortunately, careless conversation about patients is common in health care facilities. All one has to do is walk by a busy nursing station on an in-patient unit to overhear private details of patients' conditions and treatments. Patient information can be overheard on elevators transporting staff members, over lunch in the facility's cafeteria, and in other inappropriate locations. The design of most health care facilities, with semiprivate rooms, caregiver stations within earshot of waiting areas, and registration areas in main lobbies, has compounded the problem. And in teaching hospitals, traditional medical education techniques, where "teaching rounds" are conducted at bedsides and in hallways, make every detail of the patient's condition fair game for anyone nearby. Obviously, caregivers must exchange information to perform effectively as a team, but often there are few private areas for accomplishing this safely.

### Accessing Information on Cases in Which You Are Not Involved

If your system permits employees to look up information about all patients—not just the patients for whom they are caring—you should anticipate that they will. Taylor and Kitson (1995) reported on a large Michigan hospital with extensive computerized patient information available via terminals that surveyed their employees to determine whether those employees were inappropriately accessing patient information. Key staff were concerned that employees might be browsing through computerized files to which they shouldn't have access. As the first step in determining whether inappropriate access was taking place, all employees were asked to report anonymously whether they had ever used the computer to look up patient information inappropriately. Almost 10 percent of the employees were willing to admit that they had done that. Fifteen percent of respondents reported that although they hadn't done that, they had seen a coworker do it. Employees reported looking up information on family members, public figures and celebrities, and coworkers.

As Taylor and Kitson noted, the problem of unauthorized access appeared to be slightly greater with the computerized medical record than with the paper-based record: Whereas 15.5 percent of the respondents reported witnessing unauthorized computer access of patient information, only 11.1 percent reported witnessing unauthorized reading of paper files.

This hospital's results were far better, however, than the results reported by Curran and Curran (1991) in a study at a large Southern hospital. That employee survey found that 72 percent of respondents admitted to obtaining information about patients outside their assigned clinical area.

### Gossip Outside the Workplace

It isn't unusual for people to talk about their workplace with a spouse, family member, and friends. One of the first questions that greets many of us as we walk through the door at the end of each workday is, "How was your day?" The problem for health care providers is that discussions about the workplace have the potential to jeopardize patient confidentiality. This problem can be especially problematic in smaller communities, where family members and friends may be curious about the condition of patients they know.

Often, confidentiality training in health care facilities discusses the need for discretion in the workplace but fails to address how to handle requests for information that come from friends, family, and neighbors. And in physician practices and small clinics, confidentiality training often does not occur.

A study by Ullom-Minnich and Kallail (1993) examined strategies used by physicians to safeguard confidentiality in small communities in Kansas and found that the risks to confidentiality can magnify in small, tightly knit communities. In the smallest communities of under five thousand population, 14 percent of the responding physicians indicated that they had experienced instances in which patient information had passed through the physician office to an outside party who knew the patient in question, whereas in communities of over twenty thousand population, only 6 percent of the physicians agreed that this had occurred. It is interesting that only eleven of the 510 participating physicians reported that their office had strict firing policies for employees who breached patient confidentiality.

Regardless of the care setting, policies should make clear that divulging patient information without authorization, whether well-intentioned or not, is prohibited except under very limited circumstances. Those circumstances are discussed in Chapters Four and Five.

### Careless Handling and Disposal of Information

A quick glance through your facility's wastebaskets can yield some surprising information about your organization and its patients. If staff are disposing of copies of confidential information and reports without first rendering them unreadable, such as by shredding, you may be risking a breach of confidentiality. Confidential information might need to be disposed of for many reasons, including

- The state-specified retention period for that information has expired.

- The information is being microfilmed or imaged and hard copies are no longer required.

- Staff have printed out hard copies of electronic information for convenience in discussing the information at a meeting, but it is no longer needed.

In some cases, actual destruction might be taking place off-site, such as when paper records have been sent off-site to a microfilming or imaging vendor. Many such vendors have secure facilities and well-defined destruction procedures, but this is certainly an area to address in contract language with the vendor.

The growth of paper recycling programs in health care facilities has posed some additional destruction-related risks. If confidential information is collected from throughout your facility, are the collection points secure? Who has access to the collection bins? How are the bins combined, and who does this? Is shredding done before the paper leaves the facility, or are the bins transported off-site for shredding and pulverizing? Are intermediate stops made? If so, who would have access to the paper before it is destroyed? Does the facility have a written contract with the recycling company that addresses the confidentiality-related obligations of the recycling vendor's staff and drivers? By what method is the paper rendered unreadable? The American Health Information Management Association's recommendations for contract provisions to consider with vendors involved in record destruction can be found in Figure 3.1.

## RECENTLY REPORTED CONFIDENTIALITY BREACHES

A few recently published stories on privacy and confidentiality illustrate just how easy it is for confidentiality to be breached, not always with the intention to harm.

**Figure 3.1. Contracts for Destruction of Patient Records/Information.**

---

If destruction services are contracted, the contract should

- Specify the method of destruction
- Specify the time that will elapse between acquisition and destruction of data
- Establish safeguards against breaches in confidentiality
- Indemnify the health care facility from loss due to unauthorized disclosure
- Provide proof of destruction (for example, such as a certificate of destruction)

---

*Source:* American Health Information Management Association Practice Brief: *Destruction of Patient Health Information,* Chicago: AHIMA, January 1996.

- Hospitals in New York (*In Confidence*, July 1994, p. 9) and Illinois made the news when patient information was accidentally put out in the trash.

- The daughter of a Florida hospital employee had access to patient information when she visited her mother at work. She made prank phone calls to recently treated emergency department patients to tell them their HIV test results had come back as positive (*San Francisco Chronicle*, March 1, 1995, p. A2).

- A study of five Pittsburgh hospitals found that doctors routinely discussed confidential patient information in elevators, even in the presence of strangers (*San Francisco Chronicle*, July 4, 1995, p. A8).

- A physician faced disciplinary action by Connecticut health officials after informing the mother of a twenty-three-year-old patient that her daughter was using birth control. He acknowledged that the patient had not authorized him to release the information (Hladky, 1995, p. A1).

- Two hospital security guards were arrested for stealing desktop computers containing the records of several thousand patients receiving services at the South Florida AIDS network at Jackson Memorial Hospital. One of the computers was sold to an unsuspecting buyer; the other was in use at the home of one of the guards. The guards claimed they did not know what was on the computers (*In Confidence*, March 1994, p. 6).

Is it reasonable to assume that your organization is somehow immune? Can you afford to believe that these problems could not happen in your workplace?

## HOW DO YOU KNOW WHETHER YOU HAVE A PROBLEM?

There are several ways to help determine the extent of the confidentiality problems in your organization.

*Employee surveys,* such as the one described earlier in the chapter, can provide employee input. But often, even employees who understand the organization's confidentiality policies may not recognize their own actions as being problematic. For example, the well-meaning nurse who looks up her brother's pathology report after surgery may not perceive her actions as inappropriate, because her motives are "pure." Nevertheless, she has breached her brother's confidentiality.

*Incident reports and claims data* may indicate confidentiality- and privacy-related problems if those events have led to complaints or actual litigation. From what areas of your organization have the problems arisen? Can trends be seen?

*Guest relations or patient ombudsman program data* can identify patient concerns relative to confidentiality and privacy matters. Staff in these programs can be trained to ask about any concerns about privacy during patient rounds as a way of soliciting any such concerns.

*Patient satisfaction surveys* may also generate information about confidentiality- and privacy-related concerns. Many of the commercially available surveys include confidentiality-related questions. In fact, a study by one of the leading health care satisfaction survey firms reported that hospital staffs' concern for patients' privacy was one of the most significant factors in determining patients' satisfaction with their hospital experience (Press, Ganey Associates, 1992).

*Risk assessments* can be extremely useful in identifying dangerous information-handling practices. One of the important benefits of doing a risk assessment is that it attempts to identify potential problems before they become actual problems.

## THE RISK ASSESSMENT: WHY DO IT?

Unless your organization has been involved in a publicized breach of confidentiality or security, it's sometimes difficult to obtain top management's backing to spend the time and resources necessary to assess fully the risks in your health information systems. We sometimes assume that if we haven't experienced a breach of confidentiality or an information security problem, our systems are basically sound. The truth of the matter, however, is that all systems have their weaknesses. And if we haven't yet discovered our own information-handling vulnerabilities, it may be more a matter of luck than good system design.

The proposed rule on information security recently published by the Health Care Financing Administration (HCFA) will mandate risk assessments in all health care organizations that maintain electronic patient information. However, performing a risk assessment is as appropriate in paper-based organizations as in facilities with computerized health information systems. There are several compelling reasons to assess risks in our health information systems:

### Preventing the Information Disaster

Disaster prevention and business resumption planning are simply good business. Fire, flood, catastrophic power loss—all of these can threaten your organization's ability to collect, process, and retrieve data. Understanding potential disaster risks is an important part of an information system risk assessment whether your systems are computerized, paper-based, or a combination of both.

### Preventing the Confidentiality Breach

Prevention of the confidentiality breach is another reason for doing a risk assessment. Every time you read a news story about a confidentiality breach, consider whether this could happen in your organization. Asking the question is a way of keeping confidentiality and information security issues on the front burner and helps make the case for a formal risk assessment.

### Preventing Public Image Problems

Preventing public image problems is a reason for doing a risk assessment that escapes a lot of organizations until they go through a very public, and a very embarrassing, breach of security or confidentiality.

As many health care organizations have learned the hard way, patients are less likely to want to use your facility if they don't believe their privacy will be protected.

## Preventing Monetary Loss

Monetary losses from a breach of confidentiality or security can take several forms:

- Lost business

- Defense costs

- Claim payouts and settlements

- Court judgments

In considering the choice between spending a few thousand dollars in staff time doing a formal risk assessment versus spending potentially ten to twenty times more than that amount defending a lawsuit, the logic of trying to assess health information system risks becomes clear.

## THE RISK ASSESSMENT: HOW?

Once you've made the decision to assess the risks in your health information systems, what types of risks should be examined in the course of that assessment?

To be comprehensive, a confidentiality and information security risk assessment should probably include at least the following major areas of risk:

- Organizational climate risks

    Management styles and culture

    Policies and procedures

- Technology risks

    Hardware risks

    Software risks

- Environment risks

    Utility infrastructure

    Weather

- Human factors risks

    Training and education issues

    Enforcement issues

Once HCFA's final rule on security standards is published, it may serve as a good outline for organizing the internal risk assessment. See Figures 2.2 through 2.4 in Chapter Two for the categories in the proposed rule. A sample risk assessment protocol can be found in the Appendix.

# Developing Confidentiality Policies and Procedures

The federal laws, rules, and regulations discussed in Chapter Three, along with your own state's particular laws and regulations, should form the basis for detailed policies and procedures to guide staff behavior when handling, using, and disclosing confidential information. This chapter discusses issues and risks to consider when developing those policies and procedures.

First, we'll cover general principles of information release. Second, we'll examine issues related to different types of *information users*. Third, we'll examine policy and procedural issues related to various types of *information technology*.

Some samples are included to give you a head start in developing policies and procedures that make sense for your workplace. Remember, though, generic policies and procedures are not likely to meet your staff's needs for state-specific information. Your organization's health information manager can assist in tailoring generic policies into something that meets the applicable requirements.

## GENERAL PRINCIPLES OF INFORMATION RELEASE

Health care providers are bound by various laws and ethical standards to maintain the confidentiality of health information. How do we meet that obligation while facilitating the appropriate uses of that information? An understanding of some fundamental principles can help guide our actions as we consider requests for information access.

First, as noted by Brandt (1993), *it is generally agreed that the health care provider owns the physical health records, but that the patient has an ownership interest in the information* contained within those records. In other words, although the provider exercises control over the paper or digital media upon which the information is stored, the patient has certain rights to control the flow of that information. As already explained, the extent of the patient's rights may vary from state to state at present, because the recently proposed federal privacy rule does not preempt stricter state laws or regulations.

Second, *not all information that may be contained in the medical record is necessarily confidential.* For example, the date of a patient's admission to a general acute care hospital is not confidential;[10] neither is the patient's payer source. However, caution should always be exercised in releasing patient-identifiable information. In sorting out confidential information from nonconfidential information, the following questions can be useful:

1. *Is there a patient-provider relationship?* The patient and provider must have a professional relationship. What one tells the physician next door is not confidential—unless that neighbor happens to be your physician.

2. *Was the information in question exchanged through (or in the context of) the professional relationship?* The information does not have to be related verbally but could be observed by the provider or gained through physical examination, test, or procedure.

3. *Is the information needed to treat or diagnose the patient?* Data about the next of kin or the patient's date of birth are not ordinarily needed to treat or diagnose. But in some circumstances, such as mental health counseling, information about family relationships may well be needed to treat the patient and would, therefore, be confidential.

For the information in question to be considered confidential, all three questions should be answered affirmatively (Abdelhak, Grostick, Hanken, and Jacobs, 1996, p. 370).

Third, *only trained staff should be involved in the release of health information*. This helps ensure compliance with applicable laws, rules, regulations, and organizational policy.

Fourth, *any written authorization for release of information should comply with applicable state and federal laws*. In most cases, health care organizations have adopted the elements listed in Chapter Two, which describes authorizations for release of substance abuse information. This is likely to change, however, to mirror the model authorization content recommended by the federal privacy rule. See Figure 4.1 for the Model Authorization Form suggested in the proposed final rule.

Fifth, *any written authorization for release of health information should be signed by the patient or his or her legal representative or guardian*. Remember that under the proposed privacy rule, there will be no need to obtain written authorization from the patient for many types of disclosures. However, when a written authorization *is* required, patients should ordinarily sign for themselves, as long as they are competent adults or emancipated or mature minors. In the case of a minor child, the parent or legal guardian should sign. In the case of a deceased patient, the executor of the estate or an individual appointed by the probate court should sign.

If patients are incompetent, or simply unable to sign an authorization for disclosure (for example, a critically ill or unconscious patient), state laws control who may sign in their stead. The following is a typical order of priority: (1) legal guardian; (2) agent named in any advance directive, durable power of attorney for health care, or other durable power of attorney; (3) next of kin, generally in the following order: spouse, adult child, father or mother, adult brothers or sisters.

Sixth, *the authorization, when one is required, should be dated sometime following the patient's admission or outpatient encounter*. This is a common problem and source of much misunderstanding. But think about the purpose of obtaining a written authorization in the first place: It is so that the patient can make an informed decision about the disclosure of that information. Can the patient make a truly informed decision if he is signing an authorization for information that does not yet even exist? Prospective authorizations were

# Figure 4.1. Authorization for Release of Information.

**Section A: Must be completed for all authorizations**

I hereby authorize the use or disclosure of my individually identifiable health information as described below. I understand that this authorization is voluntary. I understand that if the organization authorized to receive the information is not a health plan or health care provider, the released information may no longer be protected by federal privacy regulations.

Patient name: _____ ID Number _____

Persons/organizations providing the information:

Persons/organizations receiving the information:

_____

_____

_____

_____

Specific description of information (including dates(s)):

_____

_____

_____

_____

**Section B: Must abe completed only if a health plan or a health care provider has requested the authorization**

1. The health plan or health care provider must complete the following:
   a. What is the purpose of the use or disclosure?: _____
   b. Will the health plan or health care provider requesting the authorization receive financial or in-kind compensation in exchange for using or disclosing the health information described above?                                     Yes ___ No ___
2. The patient or the patient's representative must read and initial the following statements:
   a. I understand that my health care and the payment for my health care will not be affected if I do not sign this.                                     Initials: ___
   b. I understand that I may see and copy the information described on this form if I ask for it, and that I get a copy of this form after I sign it.                                     Initials: ___

**Section C: Must be completed for all authorizations**

**The patient or the patient's representative must read and initial the following statements:**

1. I understand that this authorization will expire on __ __ / __ __ / __ __ __ __ /
   (DD/MM/YR)                                     Initials: ___
2. I understand that I may revoke this authorization at any time by notifying the providing organization in writing, but if I do it won't have any affect on any actions they took before they received the revocation.                                     Initials: ___

_____          _____
Signature of patient or patient's representative          Date
*(Form MUST be completed before signing.)*
**Printed name of patient's representative:** _____
**Relationship to the patient:** _____
                    **\* YOU MAY REFUSE TO SIGN THIS AUTHORIZATION \***
You may not use this form to release information for treatment or payment except when the information to be released is psychotherapy notes or certain research information.

*Source:* Reprinted from *Federal Register,* November 3, 1999, volume 64, number 212, p. 60065.

commonly used in the past for billing purposes. Now that the authorizations are no longer required to release information for billing purposes, the use of prospective authorizations should be sharply curtailed or even eliminated. Using a prospective authorization is potentially dangerous, as it may result in unintended disclosures—or disclosures that go well beyond what the patient desired.[11] To be safe, most health care organizations should insist upon authorizations that are signed *after* the information being requested was created.

The seventh general principle to keep in mind is that *authorizations may be revoked.* Brandt (1993, p. 8) suggests that revocations of authorization be submitted in writing to the health care provider and maintained with the patient's health record. If written revocation is impossible, an oral revocation may be accepted and should be documented by the staff member accepting it. Keep in mind that a revocation does not invalidate any releases of health information made prior to receiving the revocation. The proposed privacy rule also permits revocation of authorizations previously granted, except to the extent that the health care provider or custodian of the information has already taken action on reliance of that authorization (§164.508[e]).

With those principles in mind, let's examine the typical information disclosure practices associated with various types of common user requests. Remember that your state may have specific laws on the subject that may vary from these general practices. Also keep in mind that under the proposed federal privacy rule, even when an authorization is not required (as is the case for disclosures for treatment, payment, and health care operations), there is an exception for psychotherapy notes and research information unrelated to treatment. These items require patient authorization prior to any disclosure.


## WRITING POLICIES AND PROCEDURES FOR VARIOUS INFORMATION USERS

*Accreditation and licensing survey teams.* Surveyors may have access to patient health information to the extent required to assess compliance with applicable standards or regulations. This is often considered to be simply a part of the facility's internal quality improvement program or a normal part of health care operations. Patient authorization has not ordinarily been required in the past and is not expected to be required under the final federal privacy rule (and, indeed, is not required in the proposed rule). However, the patient-identifiable information (such as patient names) should not ordinarily leave the facility with the surveyors or appear in survey reports available outside the facility.

*Attorney (for the patient or other parties).* Written patient authorization or a valid subpoena is required prior to disclosure.

*Attorney (for your own organization).* Written patient authorization is generally not required. In-house or retained counsel are often involved in reviewing serious incidents or in preparing a defense against claims of negligence. There should be, however, a valid business purpose for the disclosure; for example, an incident being reviewed or a case pending. Under the proposed federal privacy rule, your facility's own attorney would most likely have access to protected health information for uses falling under the definition of *health care operations.*

*Courts and law enforcement.* Valid subpoenas and court orders issued by a court with proper jurisdiction should be honored and in most cases do not require a separate written authorization from the patient. However, this varies from state to state, so consult these requirements before writing facility policy. Note also that information about alcohol and substance abuse may not be disclosed without a separate court order and can only be granted after a showing of "good cause" for the disclosure. Exercise caution in responding to a subpoena for health information. If irregularities are present or there is some conflict with state or federal law (such as the substance abuse regulations), the facility should work with its attorney to file a motion to quash (that is, set aside) the subpoena.

Under the proposed federal privacy rule (§164.510 [d] and [f]), no patient authorization is required for disclosures to law enforcement officials pursuant to a legal process (such as a warrant, subpoena, or order issued by a finding of the judicial officer, grand jury subpoena, or administrative subpoena or summons or civil investigative demand) as long as that information is relevant and material to a legitimate law enforcement inquiry, the request is as specific and narrowly drawn as is reasonably practicable, and the need for information cannot be satisfied by de-identified information. With regard to disclosures for judicial and administrative proceedings, no authorization is required to disclose in response to a court order or administrative tribunal order or in any proceeding where the patient is a party and his or her medial condition or history is at issue and the disclosure is pursuant to lawful process or otherwise authorized by law.

The section of the proposed federal privacy rule on disclosure to law enforcement is highly controversial among privacy proponents, who feel that the rule will be subject to much abuse.

*Employers.* With a growing trend toward self-insuring and managing their health benefit programs, employers more frequently request health information on their employees. Written authorization of the patient has, in the past, been required before releasing health information to the employer unless the release is specifically authorized by state law, such as workers' compensation statutes. This holds true under the proposed federal privacy rule in only certain circumstances: disclosures to employers for use in employment determinations, and disclosures *prior to the patient's enrollment in a health plan* to an employer-owned health plan for making eligibility or enrollment determinations or for underwriting or risk-rating determinations. However, disclosures to employers who are directly responsible for paying the health care bill (for example, self-insured employers) would not require patient authorization.

*Family of the patient.* Contrary to many health care providers' instincts, family members are not automatically entitled to the adult patient's health information. Authorization of the patient is required if the patient is capable of making and expressing that decision (however, under the proposed federal privacy rule, a verbal indication is sufficient, and a written authorization is not required).

If the patient is incapacitated, the health care provider or plan must use some judgment, as the proposed federal rule would permit the disclosure to next-of-kin, other family member, or close personal friend but would limit the disclosure to only that which is directly relevant to the recipient's involvement in the patient's health care, consistent with good practices and ethics.

As a practical matter, patients should be queried by their care providers about their preferences for sharing information with family members, and those preferences should be clearly documented in the medical record.

*Funeral homes, coroners, medical examiners.* Requests from funeral homes generally are made in states in which funeral homes complete the death certificate. In such cases, the time and cause of death and the name and address of the attending physician may be disclosed to the funeral home without written authorization from the patient's representative. Under the proposed federal privacy rule, disclosures to coroners or medical examiners for the purposes of identifying a deceased person or determining cause of death do not require any authorization.

*Government oversight agencies and public health departments.* Many health-related agencies have the authority to access patients' health information without authorization. For example, city, county, or state health departments may have mandatory reporting of certain types of communicable diseases or some types of injuries (for example, gunshot wounds, suspected abuse). Your policies need to take into account local and state laws defining the agencies' scope of authority. Information within the scope of the requesting agency's authority can be released to legitimate representatives of these agencies. When questions arise, require the requesting agency representative to provide proof of their authority to collect the information being requested.

The proposed federal privacy rule generally permits disclosures without authorization to oversight agencies and public health authorities, and those disclosures are not subject to the "minimum necessary" standard. In other words, at this point in the rule-making process, those agencies are free to request any or all health information about any patient.

*Health care providers and employees or agents in your organization.* Some of your organization's employees and agents will need to have access to patient information in order to do their job. Patient authorization is not required to permit these employees and agents to have information on the patients for whom they are providing care or services. However, just because employees or agents are health care providers does not automatically entitle them to view information on patients for whom they are not providing services. Your policies and procedures should make it clear that employees, agents, and providers may access only the information they need to know to perform their duties (that is, in compliance with the "minimum necessary" standard). The access procedures should take into account any quality review or quality improvement responsibilities the employee or staff member has. Many organizations require employees to sign confidentiality agreements. Access controls should be in place to restrict employees and agents from browsing through the paper or electronic records of patients in whose care they are not participating. Disclosures should be on a "need to know" basis.

*Health care providers (outside your organization).* In the past, disclosures outside the organization generally required patient authorization. Exceptions could be made in emergency care situations, such as when a former patient has been taken to another facility's emergency department (and time or circumstances do not permit authorization to be obtained) or when directly transferring a patient to another health care organization for continued care.

The requirement for authorization has been eroding for some time now. Federal law, the Emergency Treatment and Labor Act, requires the transferring health care facility to send copies of relevant medical records to the receiving facility so that care can be continued. Medicare's conditions of participation also require the sending of medical records when a patient is being transferred from a hospital to a nursing facility.

Under the newly proposed federal privacy rule, disclosures for treatment purposes do not require patient authorization—even if the disclosure is being made outside your own organization (for example, to a physician in another city). As long as the disclosure is being made for treatment purposes, no authorization is required, but the "minimum necessary" standard does apply.

*Insurers and payers.* This area will change dramatically under the proposed federal privacy rule. Written authorization will no longer be required for information disclosures for payment purposes. Patients will have the option to request restricting the flow of their information to the insurer (most likely in circumstances where the patient wishes to be financially responsible for the bill), but health care providers and plans are not bound to agree to those requests.

Probably the most practical way to make the best of this situation is to make it clear to patients, before treatment, that their information will be released to their insurer if they wish the insurer to be billed. If the patient objects to this release of information, the patient can make other arrangements to pay the bill. This is the approach anticipated by some bills recently considered by Congress (for example, S. 573, the Medical Information Privacy and Security Act, and S. 578, the Health Care Personal Information Nondisclosure Act of 1999). Workers' compensation carriers have special authority in many states to access patient information without authorization. In developing your policy for handling workers' compensation requests for information, refer to state laws.

*News media.* Patient information should not be released to the news media without patient authorization under almost all circumstances. Courts have held, however, that when the patient is a public figure, the person's right to privacy should be weighed against the public's right to know. Balancing that need can be difficult and has resulted in most facilities agreeing to release only the most basic information (such as directory information) about public figures: confirming admission and their condition (for example, good, fair, poor, critical) but not releasing any further details without the patient's authorization. (Remember, though, that for substance abuse treatment facilities, the mere fact of confirming admission is a breach of confidentiality.) When public figures and celebrities are being treated, consideration may need to be given to using special security procedures for their health information to help prevent "leaks." Some facilities use separate filing systems for paper records or special high-security access codes for a celebrity's electronic health records. Procedures suggested by the American Health Information Management Association can be found in the Appendix under "Resources."

When a patient is incapacitated and therefore incapable of authorizing the release of directory information to the press, a health care provider may, at its discretion and consistent with good medical practice and any prior expressions of preference of which the organization is aware, disclose health information for directory purposes.

*Patients, residents, and clients.* Many but not all states currently permit patients or their legal representatives to review and obtain copies of the patients' health information from hospital care. Some states place limits on that access, such as only after completion of treatment, or in the case of psychiatric records, only if the physician agrees that the release would not be harmful. Fewer states speak to patients' right to review and copy their physician office record. The proposed federal privacy rule would permit patients to access their health information but only covers that portion of the patients' medical records that is maintained electronically or that is electronically transmitted. Until that issue is resolved by federal legislation or a change in the final privacy rules, your policies should reflect all applicable laws.

Whatever degree of access the laws permit, your policies should require basic security precautions before information is released to patients. For example, care should be taken to identify reliably the person claiming to be the former patient. In addition, if on-site record review is being requested instead of copies, that review should be supervised to guard against alterations or destruction of the information. If patients wish to review their health information during treatment, it is generally wise to discuss that request with their physicians or care providers, who should be encouraged to review the information with the patients and answer questions.

*Quality review and improvement committee members.* Patient information is vitally important as a data source for quality-improvement activities. Members of committees charged with legitimate quality review functions may be permitted access to relevant patient information within the committee's purview, without patient authorization. However, it is unwise to turn records automatically over to someone simply because he or she happens to be on a committee. Facility policies should require that when a committee member requests to review the records of patients in whose care he or she is not involved, the purpose of the request is verified. Suspicious requests should be referred to the department or committee chairman. Keep in mind, as well, that these internal disclosures are subject to the "minimum necessary" standard.

*Researchers.* Research projects approved by an institutional review board may generally use patient information without obtaining patient authorization. However, the proposed federal privacy rule imposes certain criteria that must be met by the researchers requesting access to information, such as a "waiver of authorization" approved by an institutional review board operating in compliance with federal regulations, or a privacy board made up of members competent in the area being researched and that includes at least one member who is not affiliated with the entity conducting the research and no members having a conflict of interest with the research. This waiver of authorization must be dated and meet numerous criteria specified in the proposed privacy rule (see 164.510[j][3]). One of those criteria that must be met is a showing that the research could not practicably be conducted without access to protected health information.

Even if the criteria are met, the research protocol should be reviewed to ensure that adequate protections are in place for that information, once it is released. Often, research needs can be met without disclosing patient-identifiable information such as name. This should be considered as research requests are received, so only the information that is absolutely necessary is disclosed. Projects that require the researchers to contact patients directly can be problematic, because in many circumstances, the act of verifying whether a patient is part of a specific group (for example, asthma patients) is, in itself, a disclosure of protected confidential information. Health care facilities that wish to participate in the research project but do not see a need to disclose patient identities and addresses sometimes avoid that problem by acting as an intermediary, contacting the selected patients to notify them of the planned research and giving them the option to participate. The addresses of those patients who agree to participate are then shared with the research team.

*Students and releases for educational uses.* Patient information can be a valuable teaching tool. To the extent possible, patient identities should be masked when information is used in case summaries, presentations, videotapes, and photographs for educational purposes. Valid internal educational uses of patient information do not require patient authorization (and would be considered a normal part of health care operations under the proposed federal privacy rule), but there should be procedures in place to verify the validity of a student's request for patient information. It is also wise to include, in any contracts with schools and universities supplying students and instructors to your facility, a requirement for students and instructors to follow your organization's confidentiality and information security policies. This is likely to be mandated under the proposed information security standards. Many health care organizations require students to sign confidentiality agreements, as well.

## POLICY AND PROCEDURAL ISSUES FOR VARIOUS TECHNOLOGIES

In developing your organization's policies and procedures for information storage and release, it is important to consider some of the special risks presented by various types of information technology; for example, electronic records, fax machines, e-mail, telemedicine, telephones and voice-mail, and the like. This section discusses some of the common technologies in use for maintaining, transferring, and disclosing patient information and special risks to consider when developing your organization's policies.

### Computerized Patient Information (Desktop, Network, Handheld, Portable)

Putting patient information onto computers offers many benefits, but it also presents some risks. Perhaps a useful way of anticipating those risks is to classify them into hardware-related, software-related, environment-related, and human-related risks.

*Hardware-Related Risks.* What sort of hardware-related risks are out there? One that appears to be poorly controlled is the risk of *theft or physical loss.* This risk is growing—especially in home health and community-based programs where handheld computers and laptops are going out into the community with caregivers. Do staff always keep the hardware with them, or does it get left out on the car seat, an attractive target to passers-by? But the risk isn't limited to transporting the hardware in cars. Many facilities have had desktop computers stolen from unlocked and locked offices and have had laptops with confidential information on them left in restaurants and stolen from their employees' homes.

Another hardware-related risk is the *failure to have current backups* of the systems' contents. Chances are, your network administrators have this well covered for data on the network. But what about any confidential data stored on desktop stand-alone systems, such as tumor registry, quality and risk management tracking programs, and so on? If that hardware fails or is lost, do you have a back-up system in place?

We also face risks if we lack certain policies and procedures to prevent hardware-related problems. For example, think about the issues that arise during *computer repairs.* If a desktop system's hard drive fails, who is authorized to work on the system? Does our own information systems department coordinate this? Does the affected department contact a vendor on their own? Will that vendor have access to confidential data? Does that vendor have to sign a confidentiality agreement? Under the proposed federal privacy rule and the proposed information security regulations, outside contractors and business partners with access to protected health information will be required to execute contracts obligating them to protect the confidentiality of the information they receive.

Risks can also be posed by hardware *upgrades.* In a perfect world, all system upgrades would work perfectly with what is already on our systems. But the hardware upgrades out there truly aren't all "plug and play"—even when they say they are. My own office discovered some problems in a recent (and, we thought, simple) modem upgrade that crashed our system temporarily. Now we have steps in place to have a very current backup file ready whenever we do any form of hardware upgrade.

Another risk associated with hardware is for those of us who are on the "leading edge" of technology. Someone always has to be the first one to test a new computer device or peripheral. At the risk of sounding like a technology reactionary, when it is a system that includes business-critical information such as patient information, sometimes it is better *not* to be on the "bleeding edge" of new technology. It may be worth waiting, letting someone else put new technology through its initial paces and, of course, anticipating the need for testing when new technology is brought on board.

*Data remanence* is a hardware-related and software-related risk that can have some important implications for our computerized systems. When most of us think of deleting information on our computer systems, we usually are under the impression that once deleted, the information has been permanently removed from our system and is inaccessible to others. In truth, however, that is generally not the case—and the information remaining on our systems could result in unauthorized disclosure. If you've ever used software to recover a file that you've accidentally erased, you've seen data remanence firsthand.

In the typical situation, entering a command on a PC to delete a file stored on electronic media results in directory information being changed to remove or mask references to the file, but the information itself is not immediately erased from the disk or tape. The term data *remanence* refers to the fact that information remains on the system after a user has deleted the file.

Although most mainframe operating systems include security features that can be used to prevent access to deleted files, personal computer operating systems typically do not include such safeguards. In fact, just the opposite is true—utility software designed to read and restore deleted files is widely available and widely in use on our desktop systems.

So, especially when personal computers are shared by multiple parties with varying levels of access rights to a database, simply deleting confidential files may not be sufficient to prevent unauthorized disclosure of information. See Figure 4.2 for some ideas on ways to prevent data remanence from resulting in an unintended disclosure of confidential information.

*Software-Related Risks.* There are also *software-related risks* to consider when developing policies and procedures. Following are some of the issues that tend to be most problematic.

First and perhaps foremost, we often have *inadequate access controls.* In other words, all too often, it is too easy for people *without* a legitimate "need to know" to get into our systems and peruse and manipulate patient information. The classic example is the hospital or large group practice

**Figure 4.2. Ideas on Preventing Data Remanence Problems.**

1. Don't permit, or at least carefully control, the use of file recovery utility software on shared personal computers or networks.

2. Encrypt confidential files. Even though deleted files may remain on the media, the encryption helps protect the information from unauthorized disclosure.

3. Initialize or reformat diskettes containing confidential information after the files are no longer needed.

4. Store confidential files on removable media. More and more systems are being designed with removable hard drives. Control those drives when not in use to prevent unauthorized access to the data.

5. Use utility software specifically to overwrite files that have been deleted. Software is available to write an erasure pattern on the disk to obliterate the prior information.

6. Don't place used tapes or diskettes in a common area to be made available for anyone to use. Trying to save money by sharing used diskettes may not be worth the cost of potential breaches of confidentiality.

7. Physically destroy diskettes and tapes that are being discarded.

that lets any physician access any patient's file—whether or not he or she is attending or consulting on the case. We often fall into this trap because of the logistical difficulties of quickly changing access rights in our computer system. So instead of working on the system to make it quicker to identify consultants and add their ID code to the list of approved users for a particular file, we literally throw open the system doors and let anyone have access to anything. That poses a serious risk to patient confidentiality and will violate the proposed federal privacy rule as well as the information security regulations.

Second, if you have passwords, you very likely have *password problems.* Take a walk through your facility to observe the computer workstations. Here's what you might find: the employee who tapes her password to her computer monitor, the employee who "hides" his password on the back of his keyboard, the doctor who gives his password to his practice manager so that she can go in and electronically sign his dictation, and the entire department that uses the word *password* for their password, so you can't ever tell which employee was using the computer. Can you top these examples?

Our password systems aren't perfect to begin with, but often we haven't given our employees much guidance on how to choose a good password (such as a nonsense word of six to seven characters or a combination of letters and numbers) and how (or why) to keep it a secret.

A third software-related risk issue that computers present is a breach of confidentiality from a *failure to encrypt,* or scramble, confidential data when appropriate. Encryption programs use a "key" (code or password) to scramble data to make it unreadable to all except those with the correct key or password. At the very least, when data are going outside the four walls of your facility, encryption is a very good idea (and may be required if the data will be transmitted via the Internet, according to the proposed information security regulations).

*Viruses* are a fourth software-related risk our systems face. Most viruses are simply nuisances, but viruses can do serious damage to your data and your programs. Without virus prevention strategies and detection software, you run the risk—in a best-case scenario—of having to spend a lot of time cleaning systems after a virus has been detected. In a worst-case scenario, your system could be crippled and your data destroyed.

Fifth is a somewhat related risk issue of software brought in from home computers. Can you guarantee that employees don't do this? Often this happens as a well-meaning attempt to save the organization some money, other times to load a favorite game. Home software poses at least three risks. Not only do you run the risk of viruses, you also run risks of *incompatibility problems.* In addition, it can pose a risk of liability for software *licensing violations.* Making copies of software without paying for them is stealing, unless the license agreement permits it. Make sure your employees do not load personal software onto your organization's computers without first clearing it through the information systems staff.

A sixth group of software-related risks is the *contract problems* that can arise with custom software vendors. If you contract with a vendor to write code for your health information system, who owns that code? What will happen if the vendor goes out of business? What if you choose to cancel the contract—will you still be able to use the software you've already had developed? Will your patient data be usable if you are no longer able to use this particular software?

*Environment-Related Risks.* Computers are not immune from *environment-related risks.* Here are some issues you should address when developing your own policies and procedures.

Have you anticipated the risk of power failure or brownouts—in other words, are all vital data systems protected from line and voltage problems?

What will happen if the telecommunications system fails? How will any offsite locations be affected? What contingency plans should be in place? A few years back, in about a five-square-mile area around my home, phone capabilities were completely knocked out for forty-eight hours. That included one local hospital, several dozen physician offices, numerous ambulatory care facilities, and more. Businesses were literally running by cellular phones, with employees sitting in their cars in the parking lot. What would prevent this from happening to you?

The risk of fire is one we're generally well acquainted with in health care—after all, we've been running fire drills for years. But have we ever included information-system components in those drills? What would happen if a wiring problem ignited a fire in our phone station box or the room holding our network servers? Have we ever really walked through a drill involving damage to the computer systems?

And what about flood damage? Don't think only of weather-related problems, because floods can happen anywhere. Pipes leak. Plumbing breaks. How would our information systems be protected from a flooding problem?

Most health care facilities tend to plan for weather-related problems. But very often, we've only done disaster drills in patient care areas and not really examined what risks they could pose to our infrastructure—including our information systems.

*Human-Related Risks.* The risks posed by *what people do, and what people don't do,* are probably the most likely source of problems for our information systems. People do make mistakes. We can minimize this through training, but we need to accept the fact that occasionally an honest mistake will be made. The wrong tape will be loaded, the wrong key will be pressed, a file will be deleted by mistake. Our systems need to anticipate common errors and we need to simplify our procedures continually to make it easier for employees to do the right thing.

We also have to anticipate the potential for deliberate actions, or sabotage. Are our systems vulnerable to sabotage? How do we control and limit high-level access privileges? How do we make sure that terminated or laid-off employees no longer have system access?

## E-mail and Internet Access

Both e-mail and Internet access pose some potential risks to confidentiality if used inappropriately. Some health care organizations and physician offices are already taking advantage of the convenience of e-mail to discuss test results and other confidential information with patients.

Technologically oriented patients may like this development, as it offers the convenience of avoiding the need to call in for test results or questions. The problem is that those same patients may not realize that e-mail really can't be considered to be completely confidential. It's best to think of unencrypted e-mail as an electronic postcard that can potentially be read by others (for example, systems maintenance personnel for servers along the chain of communication).

So does that mean never use e-mail to talk to patients? Not necessarily. Many times we talk to patients about nonconfidential things—scheduling preferences and so on. But sensitive information should not be discussed ordinarily via e-mail unless the patient is aware of the risks and still wishes to communicate in this way. If you do choose to use e-mail to communicate confidential information, implement the use of encryption software to mask the content of the transmission to all those who do not have the decryption key or password.

We may also run the risk of breaching confidentiality by staff participation in Internet chat groups and *listservs* (e-mailing lists of people with similar interests to discuss common problems). There are many groups and listservs that cater to health care professionals with topics ranging from anesthesia care, Joint Commission preparation, nursing care, and health care safety to risk management and hundreds more. Problems can arise when participants fail to exercise caution and discretion and divulge confidential information in the process of posing or answering a question. That information is then available to hundreds or even thousands of people. Imagine this scenario:

The chairman of the anesthesia department at a large community hospital is reviewing the intraoperative death of a seventy-two-year-old male. The patient's blood pressure dropped almost immediately after induction, and the anesthesia provider was unable to manage the situation successfully. As part of their routine mortality review, the department reviewed the care, but members disagreed on the proper management of the situation, and the chairman now wants other opinions on the case to help fairly resolve the dispute. He scans the anesthesia record into the computer and attaches the file to a message sent to the listserv, asking for opinions on the anesthesia care provided. Unfortunately, the patient's name and hospital identifiers are left on the scanned page. The file is distributed to over five hundred listserv participants, some of whom are anesthesia providers and some of whom are risk managers, quality managers, and simply lay persons with an interest in anesthesia.

Although the action was well-intentioned, a breach of confidentiality has occurred. Your policies should give guidance to your staff on the use of e-mail and the Internet, and prohibit the sharing of confidential information in public forums. See Figure 4.3 for sample policy language.

### Figure 4.3. E-Mail and Internet Policy.

Statement of purpose: To provide guidelines for the use of e-mail/Internet

Applies to: All employees, volunteers, and professional staff using XYZ organization computer facilities

I. **Policy**

A. Network and stand-alone systems and services shall be used in ways consistent with overall organization policy and in conformance with local, state, and federal laws and requirements.

B. Network and stand-alone systems and services will be used for mission-related purposes, including the carrying out of day-to-day operations.

C. Network and stand-alone systems and services shall not be used in a way that is disruptive to the operation of the organization or offensive to others.

D. Users shall adhere to policies regarding confidentiality and release of information as defined in the facility's policies on information security and release of patient information and access to medical records.

E. Confidentiality of electronic communications services cannot be guaranteed. All communications should be assumed to be unsecured. Use the postcard rule: "Don't send anything you wouldn't put on a postcard."

*(Continued)*

**Figure 4.3. Continued.**

II. **Procedures**
  A. Authorization will be granted to personnel who require access to network systems and services for reasons that include
    1. Retrieving and disseminating business-related information.
    2. Trouble-shooting hardware and software problems.
    3. Preventing unauthorized access and system misuse.
    4. Assuring compliance with software copyright and distribution policies.
  B. Confidential information shall not be transmitted or forwarded to
    1. Outside companies or individuals not authorized to receive such information.
    2. Internal users who have no business reason for such information.
  C. Health care information that identifies the patient, physician, or employee shall not be transmitted via the Internet.
  D. System users shall not attempt to gain access to any e-mail messages not addressed to them. Normal disciplinary processes related to privacy and confidentiality shall apply, up to and including termination.
  E. Use of network systems is a privilege that may be revoked at any time for inappropriate use or misconduct.
    1. All users shall be responsible for complying with the guidelines contained in this policy and human resources policy addressing ethical standards and conflicts of interest.
    2. Violation shall result in revocation of network-systems privileges and any other applicable actions described in human resources policy addressing disciplinary procedures.
  F. Monitoring will occur to ensure compliance with these policies and procedures.
  G. As technology for communication and information processing evolves, the organization will continue to examine and refine its information management policies.
  H. Users may use network and stand-alone systems to access e-mail and the following approved Internet services:
    1. World Wide Web for business-related purposes.
    2. Gopher.
    3. Telnet.

I. Internet services which are not approved for use through network and stand-alone systems include the following:
1. Newsgroups.
2. Internet relay chat (IRC).
3. Internet phone.
4. Online gaming.
5. Multi-user domain-dungeon (MUD).

Use of nonapproved Internet services shall result in revocation of network-systems access privileges and any other applicable actions described in human resources policy addressing disciplinary procedure:

J. The following guidelines apply to general Internet access:
1. Users may use the Internet for professional activities. Users may use the Internet to connect to resources that provide information relating to business-related and educational activities and participate in reading electronic mail discussion groups on professional topics.
2. Users shall conform to the standards of conduct and specific rules of etiquette when accessing the Internet. Users shall use their access to the Internet in a responsible and informed way, conforming to network etiquette and courtesies. Use of the Internet encompasses many different interconnected networks and computer systems. Many of the systems are provided free of charge by universities, public service organizations, and companies, and each system has its own rules and limitations. Specific inappropriate conduct includes but is not limited to
   a. Use of the Internet for unlawful activities.
   b. Use of the Internet for commercial activities not related to the organization.
   c. Activities that interfere with the ability of other users to use the network effectively.
   d. Violations of computer-system security.
   e. Any communication that violates any applicable laws and regulations.
   f. Violation of copyright law.
3. Users may download files from the Internet if not otherwise prohibited. These files must be scanned for a virus using an antivirus program provided by the information systems department.

*(Continued)*

**Figure 4.3. Continued.**

---

4. All users should complete training on Internet basics before using it. This includes information about e-mail; Telnet; anonymous ftp; use of listservs, mailing list, and discussion groups; use of Internet search engines; and features of Internet browsers.

5. The following guidelines apply to using e-mail:
   a. No spamming or sending of bulk e-mail.
   b. No mail bombs, flames, or similar kinds of mail.
   c. E-mail listservs or list subscriptions should be limited to those actually read. All files not read or no longer needed should be deleted.
   d. The use of broadcast mail (sending the same note to groups of employees or students) will be selectively used for compelling mission-related or business reasons only.

6. The following guidelines apply to use of the World Wide Web:
   a. Websites providing sexually explicit content shall not be visited.
   b. Use of the World Wide Web should be limited to mission-related or business reasons and should not disrupt the workplace.

7. The following guidelines apply to use of file transfer protocol (ftp):
   a. Illegal copies of software shall not be obtained.
   b. Licensed software shall not be distributed to others.
   c. Attach only to systems for which an authorized log-in has been obtained.

8. The following guidelines apply to the use of Telnet:
   a. Log-in should be limited only to those systems for which an authorized log-in has been obtained.
   b. Log-in as a "system administrator" or "supervisor" shall not be attempted unless the user is the authorized "system administrator" or "supervisor" for that system. This is considered a break-in attempt.
   c. Suspected violations of this policy and guidelines should be reported to the risk management department.

(Sample only. Not for use without review by legal counsel.)

---

## Facsimile (Fax) Machines

Fax machines have become an essential part of today's office equipment. If your organization hasn't already developed policies for what information should and should not be faxed and what steps to take in sending a fax, consider obtaining guidelines published by the American Health Information Management Association, which are summarized in Figure 4.4.

It is important that all faxes of confidential information be accompanied by a cover page. Sometimes we think of cover pages as a real waste of space and a waste of transmission time, but when sending confidential information, they serve a valuable purpose. First, you can notify the recipient that the information in the fax is confidential and may be protected by law and that they should not re-release this information to others. That notice can also give the recipient instructions on what to do if they receive the fax in error.

How many of us have ever received a fax intended for someone else? It's rather common. At a seminar sponsored by the National Computer Security

## Figure 4.4. Precautions When Faxing Health Information.

- Use fax only when original record or mail-delivered copies won't meet the needs of immediate patient care.
- Limit what is faxed to that which is required to meet the requester's needs.
- Obtain patient authorization for the disclosure, except as required by law.
- Include a cover page that contains a confidentiality notice and prohibition against redisclosure.
- Instruct the recipient to contact you if they are not the intended recipient.
- Take reasonable steps to avoid misdialing; for example, by pre-programming numbers that are used frequently.
- Locate faxes in secure areas where access is limited to appropriate staff.
- Monitor incoming documents so they can be routed immediately in a secure fashion.
- Develop steps for your staff to follow if a fax is sent to the wrong destination.

*Source:* Adapted from American Health Information Management Practice Brief, *Facsimile Transmission of Health Information,* Chicago: AHIMA, July-August 1996, p. 2.

Association (now the International Computer Security Association) a few years ago, one of the speakers reported that a Florida woman, over the course of one year, had received faxes of medical information on no fewer than sixty people, because her personal fax number is one digit off from a local physician's fax number. By putting instructions on the cover page, we at least stand a chance of that recipient not compounding the problem by discussing it with others, and we can arrange for return of that fax at our expense.

Think about where your faxes are physically located. In the middle of a hallway where the public has access to documents sitting in the output tray is not the best location—especially if there is no one assigned to monitor the tray to make sure incoming documents get to their correct destination. Often, confidential information just sits there in the tray, waiting for someone to come along and pick it up. It's a good idea to have the fax in a private place and to designate someone to be responsible for monitoring incoming documents and safely routing them to the correct person.

But what does "safe" routing mean? It probably is reasonable to require that confidential faxes be taken directly to the intended party. In a large health care organization, interoffice mail could be handled by a number of people who have no business seeing patient information. Think about that when you decide who should be responsible for monitoring and routing incoming faxes.

You should have written procedures for staff to follow in safely transmitting faxes that contain confidential information. First, because of the risks of misdirected faxes, it's important for staff to know that faxing should only be done when absolutely necessary—when there's no time for conventional mailing techniques. If there are certain destinations to which your staff frequently transmit patient information, program that number into the fax machine to avoid misdials. And for sensitive information, it's also a good idea to call ahead and notify the recipient that you're about to transmit, so that party can be ready to receive the information.

Organizational procedures should also address what needs to happen when a transmission has apparently gone to the wrong party. The party who received the fax in error should be contacted with instructions on how to return the fax to you (at your expense). You probably should make sure that all staff know whom to notify of the error, such as the risk manager. Staff need also to follow up with the party who was originally supposed to receive the information, and make sure that they get the information they are awaiting.

## Pagers (Alphanumeric and Voice)

Only a few years ago, pagers posed no risk to confidentiality at all. All they displayed was the phone number of the person placing the page. With advances in paging technology, it is now possible not only to send text messages, but also to send voice messages that can be played at the receiving end. Beyond the slight risk of misdialing and sending information to the wrong location, there is a greater risk in having that information viewed or overheard by unintended parties.

Imagine this scenario: Jane Doe calls her physician's office for the results of her most recent laboratory tests. She is particularly interested in her T-cell count, as she is undergoing treatment for AIDS. The office nurse sees that the lab report has not yet come in from the local hospital, where the test was done, although the results should have been returned by now. She knows, however, that Dr. Smith is at the hospital now, doing his morning rounds. She pages Dr. Smith with the following message: "Jane Doe's T-cell count not back yet. Stop by lab and inquire?" Unfortunately, Dr. Smith retrieves this message in the cafeteria, where he is having a quick cup of coffee with some colleagues and friends. The person sitting next to him sees the message displayed on the pager, and is surprised to learn that Jane Doe, a neighbor, has AIDS.

Staff who use pagers should be alerted to the possibility of confidentiality breaches when retrieving their messages in public areas, and staff members sending messages to pagers should be aware of the need to avoid using patient identifiers whenever possible.

## Telemedicine

Telemedicine installations are growing throughout the United States, offering some important benefits to rural and medically underserved areas. Because confidential information is being sent offsite to remote health care providers who, in some models, the patient may never even see, it is important for the patient to be aware that his or her information will be shared with others. Under the proposed federal privacy rule, however, the disclosure of information to the remote health care provider would not require written patient authorization, as long as the information is being shared for treatment purposes.

It is important to sort out information-handling and storage issues with the participating providers. Because patient information is likely to be stored at the remote site as well as the originating site, it is wise to evaluate the prospective partner's systems for preserving confidentiality before entering into telemedicine agreements. The following questions might assist in that evaluation:

- Who on the receiving end will have access to the patient information being sent?
- Is anyone in the control room besides the physician?
- Will videotapes or electronic records of the encounter be maintained?
- Will they be used for any purpose other than documentation of the treatment or diagnostic encounter (for example, teaching, marketing the telemedicine service to potential new partners)?
- Is retention of the encounter record the responsibility of the remote or the originating site?

There may also be a need for a written contract that addresses confidentiality-related issues with that remote provider if the provider falls under the definition of "business partner" within the federal privacy rule.

### Telephones, Cellular Phones, Voice Mail, and Answering Machines

When I lived in the Chicago area, I received repeated calls for a man named Dave. Dave's phone number was similar to my home number. Twice, Dave's doctor's office called my home number and left detailed messages for Dave on my voice mail. Apparently, the office staff didn't pay close enough attention to the outgoing announcement to realize that they'd misdialed. So they left me all kinds of information about Dave, including his cholesterol level, the results of his PSA (prostate) test, and whatever else they happened to do for him during his office visit.

Whenever I speak to a group on confidentiality problems, I always ask the audience to raise their hands if they have ever received a voice mail or answering machine message intended for someone else. The majority raise their hands—every time.

What should managers be telling their staff about leaving confidential information on voice mail and answering machines? Leaving confidential information on voice mail is not a good idea—even if you are sure you have reached the right number. There's no way of knowing whether that answering machine or voice mailbox is shared with others.

If the voice mail or answering machine message does seem to indicate that staff have reached the right number, the message should be limited to nonconfidential information. Perhaps Dave's doctor's staff could have said: "This is Dr. Smith's office with a message for Mr. Jones. Please call us at the office at your convenience." They could've avoided the problem if they had insisted on speaking directly to Dave.

An additional risk is posed by cellular and portable phones. Many health care providers are using cellular and cordless phones to do everything from return patient and staff phone calls to dictate full reports! The risk is that the calls can sometimes be intercepted via scanners.

When I talk about this risk to health care professionals, they often ask, "But who would do something like that?" And the answer is, unfortunately, a lot of people! Tabloid readers remember the furor in Britain a few years back, when the cellular calls of the Princess of Wales and her friend, and the Prince of Wales and his friend, were intercepted and published in the newspaper. Closer to home, we're reminded of what happened to then-Speaker of the House Newt Gingrich when his cell phone calls were intercepted and turned over to a Congressional committee investigating him.

These antics aren't limited to public figures. About a year ago, while I was speaking to a group of East Coast physicians, a psychiatrist related to me his own experience with cellular phones and scanners. While in his car on the way to the local hospital, he received an urgent phone call from a patient, forwarded by the office staff. The patient was despondent and threatening suicide. The doctor talked with the patient at length, and eventually obtained the patient's agreement to do nothing now but to come into the hospital emergency department to meet with the psychiatrist. He then terminated the call, finished the drive to the hospital, and walked inside. While walking down the main hallway, one of the biomedical technicians came up to him and said "You did a great job with that patient, Doctor!" When the psychiatrist asked the technician what he meant, the technician explained that the biomedical equipment staff were listening on a scanner when they picked up the call between the patient and the doctor.

It would be inappropriate to suggest that cellular or cordless phones never be used, but you *should* make sure your staff who use these conveniences understand the risk and how best to minimize that risk. For example, when returning a patient's call on a cell phone, why not suggest that the health care provider inform the patient that he or she is on a cellular line, and if the patient desires more confidentiality, the provider can call back when he or she gets to a more secure line? That way, the patient has some choice in the matter.

Talk to your transcription staff about whether they are receiving dictated reports over cellular lines. You may be surprised. Some physicians are dictating patient histories and physical examinations, operative reports, and discharge summaries on cell phones. Full patient identification data and confidential details are being potentially broadcast on the airwaves, available for listening ears. Although some of the newer cellular technologies claim to minimize the risk of call interception, it is likely that many health care providers in your organization are still using less secure technology.

### Videotapes, Photographs, and Digital Imaging

Patient information now takes many forms other than the traditional paper. Not only have we converted much of the text on paper into computerized files, but we've also seen the growing use of videotaping, photography, and digital imaging techniques, which result in what one might call a "multimedia" record. Because some of these formats don't always lend themselves to storage within the traditional patient record format—a folder—the information may be stored in various locations throughout a health care organization, with inconsistent security measures protecting them.

These multimedia records may be under the control of various departments and staff, some of whom may not be familiar with the principles of proper information handling. This can lead to breaches of confidentiality when the information is not adequately protected from inappropriate disclosures.

Special care needs to be taken with these records, as they are, indeed, parts of the patient medical record and fall under the same requirements as the traditional file folder record.

Not all health care uses of videotapes and photographs are necessarily confidential, however. For example, sometimes we videotape staff meetings for educational purposes. But the multimedia records that identify the patient and document care or services provided (for example, a videotape of a surgical procedure, or a photograph of injuries to a patient who has been abused) should be subject to the same level of protection afforded to traditional medical records. And release of those tapes, photos, and records should be governed by the facility's information release policies governing confidential patient information.

## WRITING POLICIES AND PROCEDURES WITH RISKS IN MIND

As you develop and refine your organization's policies and procedures for handling and disclosing health information, an understanding of the risks posed by various technologies, such as those discussed here, will result in more comprehensive and practical guidance for your staff who work with patient information. Those procedures and policies will be the foundation from which your staff training programs are developed.

The next chapter discusses the confidentiality-related training needs of various health care audiences and is supplemented by the Appendix, which outlines the many resources available to assist your organization in protecting the confidentiality of patient's information.

# Confidentiality Training

Having the types of the policies and procedures discussed in Chapter Four is important, but simply having them written down is not enough. Staff need to understand fully how those policies and procedures relate to their own job—and why it is essential that the rules be followed. Unless protecting patient privacy and confidentiality is a fundamental part of your health care organization's culture, there will always be staff who think of those policies and procedures as just another dusty manual on the shelf or as rules that only apply to other people.

Every health care organization—indeed, every company—has its own unique atmosphere or "culture." That culture is driven by many factors, starting right at the top of the organization.

About three years ago, in presenting some confidentiality training to a large west coast medical center, I was impressed to see a huge turnout among staff. Representatives were there from almost every department in the medical center, even though the training session was not considered mandatory. But in reviewing the evaluations after the session had concluded, we noted some interesting comments and questions from several of the attendees. Some asked, "Why weren't any administrators here?" Others said, "This was valuable. I don't know why my boss didn't make more of us come!"

Obviously, confidentiality is not the only concern of health care administrators. Nor is it the only concern of our employees. But what does it say to our employees when we, as leaders, ask our employees to attend training sessions on confidentiality but fail to attend them ourselves? And what does it say to our employees if confidentiality is not included as part of the mandatory training for all new staff members, volunteers, and students?

The actions of the facility's leadership and management team translate into certain attitudes among employees that can impact our confidentiality and information security measures. How can we expect our employees to take confidentiality and information security seriously if we don't?

Another hindrance to confidentiality protection in many health care organizations is what we could call the "nobody's job" syndrome. Often, when an issue crosses many departmental lines, such as is the case with confidentiality and information security, there's really no single person or group in charge of the issue. Departments may be more or less responsible for training their own employees, and the quality of that training is uncontrolled. No one is the champion of patient confidentiality. No one keeps the issue alive and on the front burner as we go about our job assignments. No one makes sure that policies are followed and that employees know how to do the right thing.

This often results in inconsistent enforcement of the rules. How unusual would it be to find an organization with stringent confidentiality and information security policies for employees of the health information management (medical records) department, with potential penalties ranging up to discharge for violations, that nonetheless gives a nursing assistant, who engages in inappropriate loose talk about patients at a departmental party, nothing more than a verbal reminder of the need to use more discretion? The danger whenever managers enforce the rules inconsistently is that any future attempts to enforce the rules are easily subject to challenge. As a result, when you do choose to invoke serious disciplinary action in egregious situations, it may not withstand that challenge.

Yet another risk that grows out of certain organizational climates is the "I'll do it tomorrow" syndrome. In most health care organizations today, we all have many responsibilities and priorities, and sometimes only the squeakiest of wheels gets our attention. Too many times, our peers don't consider confidentiality and privacy to be a high-priority issue.

As a result, we work with managers who wait weeks before notifying the information systems department of the need to discontinue computer system access for an employee who has been fired. And we find that some department heads never bother to get their employees to the confidentiality training programs that are supposed to be mandatory (and will soon be mandatory under the proposed federal privacy rule).

All these actions (and the inaction) say things to our employees. They communicate that we don't think these issues matter very much. And that can result in behavior that puts our patients' confidentiality and information security at risk.

## EMPLOYEE EDUCATION

So what should employees be taught? Ideally, they will be taught the information they need to protect patient information while performing their specific duties. The training should be customized to their needs. Certain information is applicable to all jobs within the facility—and that information can be taught in general employee orientation sessions and periodic updates. General orientation sessions should probably address the items listed in Figure 5.1.

Even employees who never work with computers and patient information need to know enough to spot problems. For example, a housekeeping employee may not need to know much about computer passwords and virus protection, but he or she will probably need to know enough to detect when paper and printouts are being disposed of via incorrect techniques; for example, when unshredded patient information is found in wastebaskets.

Because employees have varying needs for this training, it is important to supplement any generic training with department- and job-specific confidentiality and information security requirements. Employees of the health information management department will need special training on releasing information in a variety of circumstances, whereas staff training in information systems will need to focus more heavily on

**Figure 5.1. Generic Training Ideas for New Staff.**

- What is confidentiality and information security?
- Why is it important?
  To the patient?
  To the organization?
- How can confidentiality and information security be breached, and what are the implications of a breach?
  Case studies help get the employees' attention.
  Discussing what went wrong in those cases helps introduce the next subject.
  Penalties associated with breaches should be discussed.
- How can you avoid breaching confidentiality and information security?
  While caring for patients?
    —by being aware of listeners.
    —by protecting access to paper records and terminals.
  While using the telephone?
    —how to handle incoming calls for information
    —how to fax safely
    —how to leave messages appropriately
  While talking to staff, family members, and the public?
    —by knowing the patient's wishes about information-sharing
    —by not assuming that all healthcare workers have a "right" to know
  While using the computer?
    —discuss passwords, how to choose them and keep them secret
    —discuss other access controls, such as role-based access
    —discuss rules regarding taking diskettes or paperwork home
    —discuss virus protection procedures
  At the employee's own workstation?
    —by not leaving the area unattended with patient information on display
    —by positioning monitors and papers so they are not easily read by the public
    —by destroying and disposing of information techniques properly
- What should be done if you don't know how to handle a request for information?
- Who is available to answer questions about information-handling policies and procedures?
- What should be done if a breach of confidentiality or information security is suspected?
- Confidentiality and information security are everyone's job!

information security techniques such as access control, audit trails, and backup techniques.

The proposed federal privacy rules and the proposed information security regulations also speak to the need for employee training. The privacy rule requires that all members of the workforce who are likely to obtain access to protected health information must receive training in your organization's policies and procedures with respect to privacy as relevant to their job duties (see § 164.518[b] of the proposed privacy rule). That training will have to be certified by a written statement containing the date of the training and the employee's signature attesting to the fact that the employee will honor all of your privacy-related policies and procedures. That written certification will have to be signed at least once every three years.

The training requirements associated with the proposed information security regulations are even more specific, calling for "security awareness" training for all personnel—including management—on password maintenance, incident reporting, viruses, and other malicious software; periodic security reminders for employees, agents, and contractors; and education for actual computer users on viruses, the importance of monitoring log-in successes or failures, and password management. Security awareness training would be required under these proposed regulations for all employees, agents, and contractors, including customized education that is tailored to their specific information-handling responsibilities (see § 142.308 of the proposed information security regulations).

Regardless of the specifics in the final versions of these rules and regulations, all employees will need some generic training in privacy, confidentiality, and information security. A variety of methods can be used to accomplish this most basic training. Some organizations use stand-up presentations by the health information management staff or by the risk manager. Others rely on videotapes produced either internally or commercially, such as those discussed in the Appendix under "Resources." Still others use individual, interactive computer-based training with tests to document employee understanding of the basic concepts.

Whatever methods are used, it is important to be able to demonstrate that all employees have received the training appropriate for their job responsibilities and that your organization took steps to ensure their understanding. Unless some form of posttest or demonstration of competency is required, you will be uncertain of whether the employees truly know what they need to know to avoid breaching confidentiality.

## VOLUNTEER EDUCATION

If your organization benefits from a group of volunteers, you should examine their activities to determine how they encounter confidential information. Even if you have no volunteers specifically assigned to your health information management department, volunteers overhear and handle a good deal of confidential information as they move throughout departments and areas of your facility.

Even staffing an information desk with volunteers may involve access to confidential information. For example, the mere fact that a patient is in a psychiatric unit is confidential information under federal law.

Volunteers may well be acquainted with some of your organization's patients—especially in smaller cities. They need training in the importance of respecting patients' privacy. Often, people think that stopping by a friend's hospital room, or inquiring about their health as they see a friend arriving or leaving a clinic, is simply an expression of friendship and concern. Patients may, however, see those actions as intrusive and inappropriate. Volunteers need much of the same training that is given to the organization's employees, supplemented by customized training appropriate to their volunteer responsibilities. The outline in Figure 5.1 can serve as a starting point.

Often, all volunteer training is the responsibility of the director of the volunteer program. When it comes to confidentiality and information security, however, it may be better to involve subject matter experts such as the director of health information management or the risk manager. If the volunteer will be working on computers with access to patient information, you may also need to involve the information systems manager to discuss passwords and access controls. Videotaped or computer-based training on these subjects can be helpful in accommodating the unpredictable inflow of new volunteers and avoiding the scheduling difficulties associated with getting new volunteers together in the same room at the same time.

Just as with employees, it is important to check the volunteers' understanding of what they have learned. Unless you are using some form of posttest or skill-knowledge checklist, you may discover only after a mistake has been made that not all volunteers understood their training.

## VENDOR EDUCATION

Some confidentiality and information security training should extend to the vendors and contractors who work with protected health information (training that would be required under the proposed information security regulations). Vendors and contractors could include hardware and software vendors, a wide variety of consultants, staff from temporary employment agencies, microfilming companies, outside transcription and coding firms, paper recyclers, waste haulers, data warehouse vendors, and more.

The extent of the training should be matched to the extent of the vendor's access to your confidential data. The proposed federal privacy rule and information security regulations should be consulted to determine whether these contractors must be trained, and whether a written contract or chain of trust agreement for the handling of health information is necessary. As currently written, the proposed regulations will require written agreements with most, if not all, contractors with access to your patients' health information.

If you require your own employees to sign confidentiality statements, shouldn't vendor employees with access to your patients' data also sign similar statements? And you may wish to insist that vendors educate their own staff and certify to you that they have done so.

Vendor contracts should be reviewed by risk management or legal counsel to ensure that appropriate contractual safeguards are included that place an appropriate share of the legal responsibility for vendor employee training and compliance on the vendor's shoulders, rather than solely your own.

## MEDICAL STAFF EDUCATION

It's a rare health care organization that provides any training on confidentiality or information security to its medical staff, even though the medical staff may be facing new types of confidentiality risks in the form of remote dial-in access to hospital or community networks, cellular phones, communication with patients over the Internet, and so on. We often assume that our physicians know everything they need to know about confidentiality, but although they are acquainted with the principles, they may have very little understanding of the practical difficulties associated with some of the newer information technologies.

Medical practices, like other health care organizations, are facing increased demands for patient information. These practices often don't have access to the same resources and information-handling expertise available to staff in a larger organization such as a hospital. As a result, practice staff may be ill-prepared to handle many of the information requests they receive.

For example, what should the physician's practice manager be telling staff about leaving confidential information on voice mail and answering machines? What should practice staff do when patients ask to receive their test results via e-mail? If the practice has the ability to dial in to the local hospital's patient database to receive copies of ordered tests and other reports, what sort of password management schemes should the physician put into place? The confidentiality and information security training you offer your organization's physicians should, in addition to the minimum training required by the proposed privacy rule and information security regulations, acquaint the physicians with policy and procedure resources, as well as where they can go with questions such as these.

Ideas on issues to cover in physician training appear in Figure 5.2. By including issues germane to their office practice and staff, the training can be made particularly helpful. The many health care systems that own medical practices will need to include physician office staff members in

Privacy and Confidentiality of Health Information

**Figure 5.2. Generic Training Ideas for Physicians.**

- Typical ways confidentiality and information security are breached, and the implications of a breach.
  Case studies—physician office examples.
  Discussing what went wrong in those cases helps introduce the next subject.
- How can you and your office staff avoid breaching confidentiality and information security?
  While caring for patients?
    —by being aware of listeners, people in the waiting room
    —by protecting access to paper records and terminals
  While using the telephone, cell phones, and voice pagers?
    —how to handle incoming calls for information
    —how to fax safely
    —how to leave messages appropriately
    —the risks of cellular phone conversations
    —the risks of voice pagers
  While talking to staff, family members, and the public?
    —by knowing the patient's wishes about information sharing with their family
    —by not assuming that all health care workers have a "right" to know
  While using the computer?
    —discuss passwords, how to choose them and keep them secret
    —discuss rules regarding taking diskettes or paperwork home
    —discuss rules on e-mailing patient information and the risks
    —discuss virus protection procedures
    —discuss rules and steps for accessing the hospital network
  At the office employee's own workstation?
    —by not leaving the area unattended with patient information on display
    —by positioning monitors and papers so they are not easily read by the public
    —by destroying and disposing of information techniques properly
- What should be done if you don't know how to handle a request for information?
- Who is available to answer questions about information-handling policies and procedures?
- What should be done if a breach of confidentiality or information security is suspected?
- What resources are available to the physician's office staff?

the mandatory confidentiality training that will be required by the federal government. By customizing that training to include typical office-based problems, it can be made far more effective.

Once your organization begins offering confidentiality and information security training to physicians (if it has not already begun this process), it will be wise to have some documentation of the physicians' attendance at that training. In addition to the training, physicians using passwords to access your organization's computer system should probably be required to sign a confidentiality statement that includes an agreement not to share the password with others. If you are permitting your medical staff to dial into your organization's health care database from remote locations such as their office, it is wise to develop user IDs and require separate passwords for each practice staff member who will be accessing your database, rather than have a single password for the entire office staff. In this way, any suspicious or problematic access patterns can be traced back to the individual directly.

It's a rare health care organization these days that doesn't mention confidentiality in at least the new employee orientation, if not in training for volunteers, physicians, and vendors. But in many cases, current training consists of merely a few words about patients' rights, perhaps a requirement that the trainee sign a confidentiality statement, and a brief discussion of the need for discretion when handling patient records. Too often, that is both the beginning and end of the training we offer on the subject.

Even if we do provide everyone with some baseline training on confidentiality, often we trot out the same canned presentation year after year and fail to incorporate the new issues that arise as we change technology and expand our organizations beyond the traditional four walls. We assume that everyone knows about confidentiality. And we don't want to insult our staff's intelligence or imply that we don't trust them. As a result, our staff, our volunteers, our contractors, and our physicians may not fully understand all of the ways in which confidentiality can be breached—most often unintentionally. Until we begin to take confidentiality training seriously, those breaches will continue to occur.

# The Future

What will the future bring? In the short-term future, we are looking at the finalization and implementation of the federal privacy rule and the information security regulations. We've discussed many ways in which these rules and regulations will change information-handling and information-dissemination practices in our organizations.

Beyond the regulatory changes, perhaps the most obvious changes that are looming relate to technological advances. Since this book was started, at least one of the "near future" technology projections has become reality. Biometric identifiers as access controls are not only a possibility, they are also a reality for at least one U.S. hospital.

LaPorte Hospital in LaPorte, Indiana has implemented fingerprint identification technology as a way of controlling access to computerized health information. To obtain access to the computer, employees must scan their fingerprint, and the image is compared to the "official" image on file for that user. This ensures that users are actually who they claim to be, and employees are then permitted access to data they have been cleared to see (Carpenter, 1997).

Other identifiers can be used, such as retinal scans, voiceprints, face maps, and in the future—as strange as it may seem—body odor. Biometrics hold a good deal of promise as an access-control mechanism, as they may eliminate the need for employees to remember passwords and to safeguard special tokens or computer-access keys. Today, however, the technologies are still rather expensive, although costs are reportedly dropping quickly.

In addition to technological advances, the future is likely to bring more assaults on patient privacy and confidentiality. Information is the lifeblood of the health care system, and society will continue to find new ways to use, analyze, and (perhaps literally) profit from that information.

Medical supply houses and pharmaceutical firms are pursuing patients with direct marketing strategies as never before, and that requires the marketers to know the names of patients most likely to require their products. These lists of names are compiled in a variety of ways. Some methods have generated a good deal of controversy. Although patients filling out a questionnaire in exchange for a free sample of an over-the-counter asthma medication might not object to their name ending up on a list of asthma patients, how many patients would agree to their pharmacy selling information off patients' medication profiles? Many of the recent legislative proposals attempt to bar the sale of patient-identifiable information, and some would permit large monetary penalties against those persons attempting to profit from patient information.[12]

The Internet is likely to figure prominently in our professional future (as well as our personal lives). Providers have already begun to use the Internet to communicate with patients and colleagues across town and across the country, and even to back up and store their data. Will the protection schemes we are devising adequately safeguard that data from improper manipulation and use? Will we balance convenience and efficiency with patients' need for privacy? Will we continue to treat health information as our own commodity, or will we finally recognize that patients have a legitimate ownership interest in how their information is used? These issues will be with us for many years to come.

In the near-term future, we are likely to see congressional action on the confidentiality of health care information. And all of us will be heavily involved in (and expending considerable resources in) implementing the proposed privacy and information security regulations. That, if nothing else, will cause all health care providers to begin examining the security and confidentiality of their manual and electronic health information systems, and should cause a renewed interest in confidentiality within our organizations.

It would be satisfying to think that health care providers strive to protect patient confidentiality simply because it is the right thing to do. But in many organizations, we still devote few resources to educating our staff about confidentiality, and we settle for information systems that unnecessarily sacrifice privacy for our own convenience. Why does this still happen, when we all generally agree that protecting patients' confidentiality should be a goal? What will finally convince us that we must improve our information-handling practices?

Whether we commit ourselves to confidentiality or not, public interest in protecting the privacy of health information is likely to continue to grow. With each new headline trumpeting the careless handling of patients' most intimate secrets, public pressure for accountability is likely to increase. Some health care organizations are already realizing the marketing and public relations benefits of a strong commitment to confidentiality, and are publicly announcing their commitment on their websites and marketing materials. See Figure 6.1 for some examples of health care organizations' including confidentiality policies in their websites.

**Figure 6.1.  Some Health Care Organization Websites that Mention Confidentiality.**

---

[www.uams.edu/infotech/confdntl.html]—The University of Arkansas for Medical Sciences' confidentiality policy

[www.behmgmt.com/confidentiality.html]—A mental health program's description of their confidentiality protections

[www.chcs-me.org/conf.html]—Confidentiality policies of Community Health and Counseling of Maine

[www.newbeginning.net/newpage6.html]—An online psychotherapy service discusses its confidentiality protections

[http://hirs.mc.duke.edu/recserv.nsf/web/confidentiality+agreement]—Duke University Medical Center's confidentiality agreement for employees

---

Perhaps public demand, in the end, will provide the motivation we need to make patient confidentiality and privacy a true priority in our organizations—whether we work in a solo physician practice, an ambulatory surgery center, a home health agency, or a nationwide, integrated health care system. It is my hope that the tools and resources in this book (and those described in the following Appendix) will assist you in meeting the present and future challenges of protecting patient confidentiality in your organization.

# APPENDIX

There are many resources available to help you when developing confidentiality-related policies, procedures, and training programs. Knowing what is available can help avoid the need to "reinvent the wheel," but it is important that any materials used for staff education be customized to your facility's own requirements. The Appendix inventories some of those resources, which include books and pamphlets, videotapes, software, and Internet-based resources. In addition, this chapter offers a basic protocol for organizing and performing a risk assessment of your health information systems.

## A RISK ASSESSMENT PROTOCOL

Chapter Three discussed the importance of performing a risk assessment to determine your health information system's weaknesses. Ways of organizing a team to perform this assessment are discussed in this section. How do you put it together? Whom should you involve?

### Who Should Do It?

Each of the following staff members has a special perspective that can be valuable in detecting and anticipating potential risks.

The organization's health information manager is fundamental to the process. When only information systems staff are performing the risk assessment, they may have a pretty good grip on technical security risks, but they probably won't have all of the necessary insights into confidentiality risks. It is vital that health information professionals be involved on the team.

The chief information officer also needs to be involved. This person is likely to have the broad overview of any computerized system capabilities and weaknesses, and can save the risk assessment team's time in coming up with answers to technical security questions.

Ideally, caregivers should be represented. The point of care is where the "rubber meets the road" in collecting and using patient information, and they will be aware of what really occurs at the point of care. It's also helpful to have caregivers involved in risk assessment from the standpoint of obtaining staff buy-in to the fact that you have information security and confidentiality risks, as well as getting buy-in to any potential solutions to the problems you identify.

Your risk manager or legal counsel also needs to be involved. If you have in-house counsel, have them at the table. If you must rely on outside lawyers, try to have them involved in at least reviewing the results of your risk assessment. Risk managers and attorneys will understand the liability implications of the problems you uncover. Sometimes, this is the only risk that convinces senior management to take problems of information security and confidentiality as seriously as they should.

The human resources manager is also a good choice, in most cases. Much of what you will uncover in your risk assessment will point out the need for policy and procedural changes. This means changing employee behavior. It may mean devising new training programs. It may mean the need for additions to your performance appraisal tools. It may mean changes to the progressive discipline system. Having the human resources manager at the table helps facilitate these changes if they are necessary.

Patient relations staff can play an important role on your risk assessment team. They understand your patients and what concerns them. They understand public relations and can help represent the patients' interests in whatever changes you consider as a result of your work.

Your finance or patient accounting manager can also be a good candidate for the risk assessment team. He or she will have insights into potential problems with electronic data transfer to payers and intermediaries.

Of course, you also want enthusiastic people who are willing to work, so in organizing your risk assessment team, don't overlook people who are champions of confidentiality and information security simply because they aren't in these categories.

Once your team is assembled, where do you begin? How can you approach such a huge task without getting completely frustrated? You're obviously going to have to gather a lot of data about *what is*. There are a lot of ways to do this, and no one way will work best for all teams. You might want to devise or use information-gathering checklists to collect basic information on information system operations. You'll also probably need to interview key staff about the information system's capabilities and potential weaknesses. You'll very likely want to interview front-line employees about how they use the system to determine the differences between what your procedures say and what really happens. Many risk assessment teams like to include at least some direct observation of system use at the point of care to get a feel for the types of information security and confidentiality problems that come up in the course of a workday.

Don't forget about some of your internal data sources that can point toward potential problems. Incident report data may indicate that certain departments are having confidentiality-related problems. Patient relations reports may identify a trend in patient complaints about privacy in a particular department. You may have already experienced lawsuits or legal claims related to confidentiality or security problems. With your risk manager or legal counsel's help, you should review those allegations to see whether they have merit and determine what, if anything, the whole organization can learn from the event.

There are a host of outside consultants available to help identify information security and confidentiality risks. Some of the major accounting and consulting firms offer this service, and there are firms specializing in health care information systems as well.

Don't overlook the consultation you may be able to obtain through your organization's liability insurer. Many of the major insurers of health care organizations employ consultants with expertise in information systems or confidentiality who can come in as a full partner on your risk assessment team—often at no charge to your organization. They can be particularly useful in doing staff interviews, because sometimes employees are willing to say something to a stranger that they would be very reluctant to say to their supervisor.

What issues should your risk assessment address? Here are some ideas on items to include as part of your risk assessment.

### Assessing Organizational Climate

You will need to look critically at senior management's role in promoting information security and confidentiality in your organization. How do they support this issue? How is their support for confidentiality relayed to staff? Has your CEO ever communicated the importance of confidentiality, or is it left for other people to cover? Have administrators ever sat through the so-called "mandatory" confidentiality training program, or are they excused from this part of your training and orientation? Do department managers make sure that their employees attend training sessions on confidentiality and information security? Do they make sure that their employees sign confidentiality statements? And most important, how do your leaders and managers make sure that your rules are enforced consistently? If a breach of confidentiality is reported on an incident or occurrence report, how do we make sure that situation giving rise to the breach is dealt with?

If your senior managers don't take seriously confidentiality and information security, no one else will. As touchy as this issue can be, if you don't include it in your risk assessment, you are missing a real opportunity to push confidentiality and information security onto the front burner.

### Assessing Hardware-Related Risks

Here's a quick checklist of hardware-related items and processes to cover as part of your risk assessment:

- What is your process of adopting new technology? Who makes purchase decisions? Do those purchase decisions include an assessment of

**84**

potential risks inherent in the technology? Is it just one person's decision, or does a knowledgeable panel or group have to give the OK? The issues should be considered for desktop PCs as well as your networks. For example, when selecting a hardware vendor, is it a decision made on price alone, or are you factoring in risk management issues such as the availability of technical support or whether next-day replacement options are available?

- What sort of physical security do you have for your hardware? Are computer systems in locked areas or made secure with lock-down or tie-down cables?

- How do you try to prevent systems from walking out the door? And for those systems that are designed to walk out the door (for example, laptops and notebooks for the home care staff), how do you instruct users to keep their portables safe? Do they follow those rules?

- How often are critical systems backed up? Are the backup media stored off-site in a secure location? Are all systems containing patient data periodically backed up? Again, backup procedures are usually well handled for a network but often are not adequately covered in smaller settings where patient data are loaded onto freestanding desktop systems.

- Have your policies been updated to cover any new technologies or systems you've adopted recently? Have employees been notified of any policy changes?

- Have procedures been written to give employees guidance on protecting the confidentiality and security of the information they use? If you are in a hospital setting, you may feel you already have this covered, but you're likely to find problems when you start purchasing medical practices and see their procedures for release of information. Your organization and its information system are constantly changing, and your procedures need to keep up with that.

- Do you have adequate firewalls in place between outside computers and the Internet and your own network? This is a software issue as well as hardware issue, and it's becoming more complex as more of our organizations are linking to the Internet and participating in community health information networks. As part of your risk assessment, be sure to look at the barriers in place between your own systems and outside networks.

## Assessing Software-Related Risks

Here are a few software-related items to consider in your risk assessment:

- How do you limit access to only people who really need to see any given patient's information? Are there ways of defeating the system? How do you balance the need for convenient access for legitimate users and the need for confidentiality?

- What sort of rules govern your password system? Must passwords be changed? Does the system force those changes periodically? How have you taught employees to choose a password, and how have you instructed them to safeguard their password?

- What files and processes warrant encryption? Should all patient-related transmissions to remote locations be encrypted? Will the encryption key be periodically changed? Who will be responsible for notifying end users of changes in the encryption key?

- How much risk are viruses in your organization? How many computers have access to outside networks and bulletin boards? How many employees take work home on disks, work at home, and bring that information back? Do all those computers have antivirus software loaded? Has the software been kept up-to-date?

- What about personal software? How many computers in your organization have outside, unapproved software loaded onto them? Does anyone have a complete inventory of what's loaded onto your computer systems? How do you teach employees to avoid loading personal software onto your computers?

- If some personal software is going to be permitted, how do you review that software license before loading to make sure the additional copy doesn't place the facility at risk of a licensing violation? Who is in charge of reviewing the license? How have employees been notified of the need to check with this department or person first?

## Assessing Environmental Risks

How do we begin to understand the potential risks in our environment? You may wish to start by looking at which computers are protected by the emergency generator or uninterruptible power supplies—and whether all vital systems are protected. You also need to make sure that every computer has at least surge protection.

Look also at whether your fire protection systems (which were probably installed years ago) are still adequate in light of the increasing use of electronics in all areas of the facility. Are there areas that need types of fire detection and extinguishing systems different from what was originally anticipated?

What about the potential for flooding? Where do the pipes run? Which systems would be affected by a leak? Can minor physical modifications be made to minimize any risks you identify? Having the engineering staff armed with blueprints involved in a physical tour of all computer locations can be helpful in spotting risks no one ever had considered.

And take a fresh look at those disaster drills we all run over and over again. Have you included information system scenarios in those drills? Many times, no one is thinking about the potential for damage to the computer network or stand-alone personal computers.

## Assessing Human Factor Risks

Next, how do you evaluate the *human factor* risks in your information systems? Probably the best place to start is to look at the training programs you give employees on confidentiality and information security. Were they written ten years ago, before the widespread adoption of computers in each department? Have you incorporated issues and risks of new technology such as voice mail, e-mail, cell phones, and the like? Do you ever test employees after training to determine whether they understand what was taught?

Do your training programs even reach everyone? If you have a confidentiality training program that is strictly voluntary, do you know whether managers get their employees there? Do you even offer the training at times convenient to all shifts to encourage attendance?

With respect to policies and procedures, how current are they? Do you update them as you incorporate new technology? How do they get distributed to all affected departments? Do you use all of your available communication channels, such as employee newsletters, to alert staff to important procedural changes that cross departmental lines?

Once you've written policies and procedures, do you enforce them? As part of your risk assessment, you're very likely to find uneven enforcement of information security and confidentiality rules. Interviews with department managers about how they would react to a certain confidentiality breach scenario is one way of uncovering this, as is a review of actual incident reports to see how the involved managers followed up on the situation.

## Conducting a Risk Assessment

So let's say you're convinced of the need to do a risk assessment. You've identified a good team, and the team has brainstormed some of the issues you need to include. Now what? Do you really have to reinvent the wheel? The good news is that there are many resources out there to help you organize a risk assessment.

The American Health Information Management Association (AHIMA) has a number of resources to get you started, as do the Computer-Based Patient Record Institute (CPRI), the International Computer Security Association, the Joint Commission on Accreditation of Healthcare Organizations (JCAHO), and many other organizations. These resources are described in greater detail later in this chapter.

After you've gathered some useful resources, the next step is to start getting some employee input as part of your risk assessment.

## Obtaining Employee Input

Don't fall into the trap of thinking that just because a policy says that something is done a certain way, it really is done that way. Employee input can help you separate fantasy from reality, and it is vital to doing an effective risk assessment. In some situations, you may wish to give employees the opportunity to give input anonymously so that they can speak without fear of reprisal. Employee surveys are often used as a way of getting this information. But if you're going to do written surveys, make sure to leave space for employees to answer the last question: "Where do you need help?" Employees will point out problems that your risk assessment team would never imagine. Give your staff the opportunity to tell you about them.

## Using the Risk Assessment Results

At this point, you should be thinking ahead and saying, "OK, I'm going to generate a lot of information during a risk assessment. What am I going to do with that information, and how can we use the results to make change?"

If your results end up in a 150-page report submitted only to the CIO or CEO, you won't make much change. Everyone who participated should have access to the results. If you thought enough of that person to ask their opinion, you should think enough of them to tell them what you learned. The wider the distribution list, the better. After all, confidentiality and information security risks are everyone's business. Everyone who has a stake in the results should also see your results—even if they weren't directly involved in the risk assessment. For example, results could be summarized for the entire clinical staff, even though only a few clinicians actually participated in the process. Brief presentation at medical staff departmental meetings, written summaries of the key findings in the employee newsletter, a presentation at the department head meeting, a presentation for the board of directors—all of these are ways of increasing your chances of getting some positive changes made.

When presenting the results and your team's recommendations, try to prioritize the problems you detected, as well as your recommendations. You already know that there are only so many dollars out there and only so many hours in each day. You may not be able to solve all the problems you identify in your risk assessment. But by prioritizing the problems with your team, you can try to encourage the organization to focus scarce resources on the issues most likely to reduce the risks of a confidentiality or security breach.

Your team will need to decide which problems are indeed the most important and deserve attention, as well as those that may not be that important but are very easy to fix and therefore deserve some attention as well.

## The Need for Reassessment

After you've gone through a rigorous risk assessment, about the last thing you'll want to do is repeat the process again quickly. Nevertheless, your team should plan at some point to sit down again and evaluate whether the actions that were taken as a result of your recommendations have been effective in eliminating the risks you identified. Reassessment can also be a socially acceptable way of holding recalcitrant managers responsible for getting changes implemented when you are unable to get their cooperation simply because implementation is a good idea. Your reassessment should receive the same kind of publicity and distribution as your original report. It's important for everyone to see that the issue hasn't died, and that confidentiality and security continue to be an important issue for your organization.

## The Benefits

Is risk assessment a big job? It is. Will it take a lot of time? It will. But it's a fundamental step along the road toward secure health information systems. By taking an organized approach toward assessing your information system risks, you will identify problems you never knew you had. You will also achieve some level of commitment to the issues by the people you involve. This has residual benefits long after the assessment is complete, such as building stronger team relationships in dealing with information system problems. Your systems will be safer for it. Your patients' information will be safer for it. And you'll be an integral part of a team that's trained in asking all the right questions so that future problems can be avoided.

## RESOURCES

What follows are some of the available resources for improving confidentiality and privacy in your organization. Contact names and numbers are given, where available, to assist you in locating and evaluating these resources.

## Books, Pamphlets, and Print Materials

*CPRI Toolkit: Managing Information Security in Health Care,* published by Computer-Based Patient Record Institute, 4915 St. Elmo Avenue, Suite 401, Bethesda, MD 20814 [http://www.cpri.org]. Included is information on how to implement security measures and to integrate good security processes into the everyday working routines in health care organizations. For ordering information, contact CPRI at 301–657–5918.

*Faxing Safeguards: Guidelines for Transmitting Patient Information,* by Mary Brandt, published by AHIMA, 1997. This set of guidelines includes sample policies and procedures, fax cover sheets, and forms. To order, contact AHIMA at 312–233–1100.

*For the Record: Protecting Electronic Health Information,* 1997, 288 pages, 6 × 9, hardbound, ISBN 0–309-05697–7. To order, contact National Academy Press, 1–800–624–6242 or 202–334–3313. This book explores ways of protecting health information in electronic formats. It recommends steps that health care organizations can take to improve privacy and security while ensuring adequate access to information.

*Health Data in the Information Age: Use, Disclosure, and Privacy,* 1994, 257 pages, 6 × 9, hardbound, ISBN 0–309–04995–4. To order, contact National Academy Press, 1–800–624–6242 or 202–334–3313. This book is the report of a study done by an Institute of Medicine committee that examined the emergence of large health databases and their implications for use in patient care, research, public health, and other private purposes. One of the book's four chapters focuses on confidentiality and privacy of personal data, including the use of universal person-identifiers such as social security numbers.

*Health Information: Management of a Strategic Resource,* 1996, 753 pages, hardbound, ISBN 0–7216-5132–1. Published by W. B. Saunders Company. This textbook is written for health information management professionals and students and covers the gamut of issues in health information management. Several of the chapters focus on data gathering, use, retention, and disclosure in both paper-based and computer-based formats.

*HIV and Confidentiality: Guidelines for Managing Health Information Relative to HIV Infection,* by Mary D. Brandt, published by AHIMA, 1997, softbound. To order, contact AHIMA at 312–233–1100. These guidelines cover the legal issues involved in collecting, maintaining, and disclosing HIV-related information, including information on HIV-infected health care staff as well as patients. It includes sample consent forms for HIV testing as well as sample authorization forms for the disclosure of HIV information.

*In Confidence,* a bimonthly newsletter published by the American Health Information Management Association. This newsletter focuses exclusively on the confidentiality of health care information and strategies for protecting it. For ordering information, contact AHIMA at 312–233–1100.

"Position Statement of AHIMA and MTIA on Confidential Health Information and the Internet," issued January 1998 by the American Health Information Management Association and the Medical Transcription Industry Alliance, 2 pages. This position statement outlines security and confidentiality-related concerns when patient information is placed on the Internet, and the need for encryption. To obtain, contact AHIMA at 312–233–1100.

*Practice Briefs,* published by AHIMA, are available on numerous subjects related to confidentiality, privacy, and information security. Some of those subjects are listed below. To order, contact AHIMA at 312–233–1100.

*Authentication of Medical Record Entries,* March 2000, 7 pages

*Destruction of Patient Health Information,* April 2000, 2 pages

*Disaster Planning for Health Information,* May 2000, 6 pages

*Disclosure of Health Information,* October 1996, 2 pages

*Electronic Signatures,* October 1998, 7 pages

*E-mail Security,* Februrary 2000, 4 pages

*Facsimile Transmission of Health Information,* July-August 1996, 2 pages

*Information Security: A Checklist for Health Care Professionals,* January 2000, 4 pages

*Managing Health Information Relating to Infection with the Human Immunodeficiency Virus (HIV)*, May 1999, 2 pages

*Managing Multimedia Medical Records*, February 1998, 2 pages

*Patient Anonymity*, November-December 1997, 3 pages

*Patient Photography, Videotaping, and Other Imaging*, 1999, 2 pages

*Protecting Patient Information After a Closure*, March 1999, 9 pages

*Release of Information for Marketing Purposes*, January 1998, 2 pages

*Telemedical Records*, April 1997, 3 pages

*Protecting Personal Health Information: A Framework for Meeting the Challenges in a Managed Care Environment*, published by the Joint Commission on Accreditation of Healthcare Organizations and the National Committee for Quality Assurance, November 1998. This joint report offers recommendations to address the demands for health information being made by managed care organizations and others. To obtain a copy, call JCAHO's Customer Service Center at 630–792–5800 or NCQA's Customer Service Center at 202–955–5697. The report is also available via both organization's websites: [www.jcaho.org] or [www.ncqa.org].

*Release and Disclosure: Guidelines Regarding Maintenance and Disclosure of Health Information*, by Mary D. Brandt, published by AHIMA, 1997, softbound. To order, contact AHIMA at 312–233–1100. This brief guidebook offers a succinct and practical set of guidelines covering the maintenance and disclosure of health information to various parties. It includes many sample forms.

*Security and Access: Guidelines for Managing Electronic Patient Health Information*, by Sandra Fuller, published by AHIMA, 1997, softbound. To order, contact AHIMA at 312–233–1100. This compact book outlines key issues in protecting the security of electronic health information.

## Videotapes

*Confidentially Speaking*, produced by the Oregon Health Information Management Association. The Oregon association has produced two excellent

VHS videotapes on confidentiality and privacy in health care settings. The first, a fourteen-minute VHS tape done in 1992, covers confidentiality basics and how to protect confidentiality in various settings. The second VHS videotape, done in 1998, focuses more heavily on issues presented when computerizing health information. For ordering information, see the ORHIMA website at [www.orhima.org/products/products.html].

*Handle This With Care,* produced by Irongate Inc. This twelve-minute VHS video helps raise awareness of the need for confidentiality and information security. For ordering information, contact Irongate at 415–491–0910, or visit their website at [www.irongateinc.com].

## Software

*Confidentiality of Information,* published by JCAHO, is a Windows-based software package available on 3.5-inch diskettes or CD-ROM. This computer-based training program is designed to educate staff about confidentiality. For ordering information, contact JCAHO at 630–792–5800.

## Associations and Organizations

The American Health Information Management Association (AHIMA) offers numerous resources on managing confidentiality and information security; many of them are listed above. To obtain a product catalog, contact AHIMA at 233 N. Michigan Avenue, Suite 2150, Chicago, IL 60601–5519; [www.ahima.org]; or telephone 312–233–1100.

The Computer-Based Patient Record Institute (CPRI) is another good source of information on this topic. Their website offers many excellent resources, including security and education guidelines for health information systems. Contact them at [www.cpri.org] or telephone 301–657–5918.

The Health Care Information Management Systems Society (HIMSS) offers educational conferences and publications that cover issues related to information security. Contact them at 230 East Ohio Street, Suite 500, Chicago, IL 60611; [www.himss.org]; or telephone 312–664–HIMSS.

Privacy Rights Clearinghouse is a nonprofit organization committed to improving the protection of citizens' privacy, including the privacy of health information. Contact them at 5384 Linda Vista Road, #306, San Diego, CA 92110; [www.privacyrights.org]; or telephone 619–298–3396.

This list is by no means exhaustive, but it will give health care organizations a good starting point in finding useful resources to improve the confidentiality and privacy of the health care information they manage.

## Internet Resources

Website addresses tend to change with time, but these were accurate when this was written. These sites offer a wealth of resources and ideas that can help you protect confidentiality in your organization. Using a search engine with search terms of "confidentiality" and "privacy" will probably add many additional entries to this list:

[http://afis.colstate.edu/stephens/cis425/moorbib.html]. Annotated bibliography on security in health care systems.

[http://aspe.os.dhhs.gov/ncvhs/privrecs.htm]. Health privacy recommendations of the National Committee on Vital and Health Statistics.

[http://eduserv.hscer.washington.edu/bioethics/topics/confiden.html]. Overview of the ethics of confidentiality, with case studies, from the University of Washington.

[www.ahima.org]. Website of the American Health Information Management Association.

[www.arentfox.com/quickguide/businesslines/e-health_telemed/e-healthnewsalerts/licenseimplic/licenseimplic.html]. Article on telemedicine's implications for patient confidentiality.

[www.cdt.org/privacy]. The Center for Democracy and Technology's privacy issues page.

[www.cpri.org]. Website of the Computer-Based Patient Record Institute.

[www.critpath.org/msphpa/ctse.txt]. Legislative survey of state confidentiality laws.

[www.epic.org/privacy/medical]. Overview of medical record privacy news, laws, and publications by the Electronic Privacy Information Center.

[www.himss.org]. Website of the Health Care Information Management Systems Society.

[www.irongateinc.com/lawsuits/html]. Website describing lawsuits involving breach of confidentiality.

[www.jhita.org]. Website of the Joint Health Care Information Technology Alliance.

[www.medg.lcs.mit.edu/courses/6893-S95/emr-medline.html]. Medline search on electronic medical records.

[www.rmf.harvard.edu/rmLibrary/rmissues/confidentiality/index.html]. Advice on confidentiality in the medical practice from the Risk Management Foundation.

# NOTES

1. Further discussions of this story figured prominently in Boston media attention for weeks. See "Medical Protection," editorial, *Boston Globe,* March 8, 1995, p. 18, and "Computers, Confidentiality, and Health Care," advertisement, *Boston Globe,* March 17, 1995, p. 17, where Harvard Community Health Plan responded with an advertisement announcing new policies to protect computerized mental health records. See also Bass, "AG to Probe Access to Psychiatric Records," *Boston Globe,* May 18, 1996, p. 17, describing the Massachusetts attorney general's investigation of the practice of computerizing psychiatric records after critics complained that the new policies announced by the health plan were insufficient to protect privacy.

2. The relevant portion of the Hippocratic oath states: "What I may see or hear in the course of the treatment, or even outside of the treatment in regard to the life of men, which on no account one must spread abroad, I will keep to myself."

3. Number 5 of the American Hospital Association's *Patient's Bill of Rights* states in part: "The patient has the right to every consideration of his privacy concerning his own medical care program."

4. The American Health Information Management Association's 1998 *Code of Ethics* calls on health information management professionals to promote and protect the confidentiality and security of health records and health information.

5. See the federal regulations governing the confidentiality of substance abuse treatment, at 42 C.F.R., Chapter 1, Part 2, Section 2.13, Revised (1983).

6. See, *Plain Dealer Publishing Co.* v. *U.S. Dept. of Labor,* 471 F. Supp. 1023 (D.D.C. 1979); *Florida Medical Assoc., Inc.* v. *U.S. Dept. of Health, Education and Welfare,* 479 F. Supp. 1291 (M.D. Fla. 1979); and *Washington Post Co.* v. *U.S. Dept. of Health and Human Services,* 690 F. 2d 252 (D.D.C. 1982).

7. There are some disclosures that may be made without prior authorization; these are described at 5 U.S.C. §552a (b) (1977).

8. Whether or not a minor may legally sign his or her own authorizations and consents is a matter of state law and varies with the state. Likewise, the party authorized to sign in lieu of a deceased patient or incapacitated patient also varies and depends upon whether an executor or guardian has been appointed.

9. §2.31(a) and (b) of the regulations outline the exact requirements and give sample language that meets the intent of the regulations. Most substance abuse programs have adopted this sample language directly into their authorizations for release of information.

10. But note that in substance abuse treatment facilities covered by the regulations discussed in Chapter Two, even the fact of the patient's admission for treatment is confidential and may not be disclosed without patient authorization except under very limited circumstances. See Chapter Two for a more complete discussion.

11. This was precisely the issue in the *Georgia* case discussed in Chapter Three.

12. For example, in the current version of S. 578, the Health Care Personal Information Nondisclosure Act of 1999, persons violating the act with the intent to sell or use health information for commercial advantage could be fined up to $500,000 and imprisoned up to ten years, whereas offenses without this intent would be assessed much lower penalties.

# REFERENCES

Abdelhak, M., Grostick, S., Hanken, M.A., and Jacobs, E. *Health Information: Management of a Strategic Resource.* Philadelphia: Saunders, 1996.

American Health Information Management Association. *Code of Ethics.* Chicago: American Health Information Management Association, 1998.

American Hospital Association. *Patient's Bill of Rights.* Chicago: American Hospital Association, 1975.

Bass, A. "HMO Puts Confidential Records On-Line." *Boston Globe,* March 7, 1995, p. 1.

Bass, A. "AG to Probe Access to Psychiatric Records." *Boston Globe,* May 18, 1996, p. 17.

Brandt, M. *Maintenance, Disclosure, and Redisclosure of Health Information.* Chicago: American Health Information Management Association, 1993, p. 5.

Brandt, M. *Information Security—An Overview.* Practice Brief. Chicago: American Health Information Management Association, June 1996.

Carpenter, J. "Confidentiality at Your Fingertips." *In Confidence,* 1997, *5*(5).

42 C.F.R. Part 2, Subpart B, 2.12, Revised 1983.

42 C.F.R., Chapter 1, Part 2, Section 2.13, Revised 1983.

"Computer Thefts Put Confidentiality at Risk." *In Confidence,* March 1994, p. 6.

"Computers, Confidentiality, and Health Care." *Boston Globe,* March 17, 1995, p. 17.

Curran, M., and Curran, K. "The Ethics of Information." *Journal of Nursing Administration,* 1991, *21,* 47–79.

Equifax. *Harris-Equifax Consumer Privacy Survey.* Atlanta: Equifax, 1993.

*Estate of Behringer* v. *Princeton Medical Center,* 249 N.J. Super. 597, 592 A.2d 1251, 1991.

*Florida Medical Assoc. Inc.* v. *U.S. Dept. of Health, Education and Welfare.* 479 F. Supp. 1291, M.D. Fla. 1979.

Givens, B. *The Privacy Rights Handbook.* New York: Avon Books, 1997.

*Health Insurance Portability and Accountability Act* of 1996 (H.R. 3103), 104th Congress.

Hladky, G. "Doctor's Disclosure Sparks Ethical Debate." *New Haven Register,* July 19, 1995, p. A1.

"Hospital Places Patient Records Out for Trash." *In Confidence,* July 1994, p. 9.

Institute of Medicine. *Health Data in the Information Age.* Washington, D.C.: National Academy of Sciences, 1994.

Joint Commission on Accreditation of Health Care Organizations. *Management of Information Standards for Health Care Organizations.* Oakbrook Terrace, Illinois: Joint Commission on Accreditation of Health Care Organizations, 1995.

McCann, R. "Protecting the Confidentiality of Peer Review Information." *Journal of AHIMA,* 1993, *64*(12), 52.

"Medical Protection." *Boston Globe,* March 8, 1995, p. 18.

*Plain Dealer Publishing Co. v. U.S. Dept. of Labor.* 471 F. Supp. 1023, D.D.C. 1979.

Press, Ganey Associates. *The Satisfaction Report.* South Bend, Indiana: Press, Ganey Associates, 1992.

Rankin, B. "Doctor, as Patient, Wins Suit in Atlanta." *Atlanta Journal-Constitution,* March 13, 1998, p. B.

"Study Finds Disregard for Patient Confidentiality." *San Francisco Chronicle,* July 4, 1995, p. A8.

Taylor, D. K., and Kitson, J. "Behavior, Attitudes, and Knowledge About Confidentiality: A Survey of Hospital Employees." *In Confidence,* 1995, *3*(4), p. 3.

"Teenager Arrested in AIDS Phone Hoax." *San Francisco Chronicle,* March 1, 1995, p. A2.

Ullom-Minnich, P. D., and Kallail, K. J. "Physicians' Strategies for Safeguarding Confidentiality: The Influence of Community and Practice Characteristics." *The Journal of Family Practice,* May, 1993, 445–448.

5 U.S.C. §552a(b). "Freedom of Information Act." 1977.

USDHHS, *Federal Register,* 1998, 63(155), 43241–43280.

USDHHS, *Federal Register,* 1999, 64(212), 59918-60065.

*Washington Post Co. v. U.S. Dept. of Health and Human Services.* 690 F. 2d 252, D.D.C. 1982.

# INDEX

## A

Abdelhak, M., 36
Access: biometric identifiers for controlling, 77; controlling, to computerized health information, 5, 25–26, 27, 50–51, 77; "least privilege" principle for permitting, 26; as presenting problems in protecting confidentiality, 4–5. *See also* Health information releases/disclosures
Accreditation and licensing survey teams, information policies and procedures for, 39–40
Accreditation standards, on confidentiality of health information, 9
Alcohol abuse records. *See* Substance abuse records
American Health Information Management Association (AHIMA), 20, 88; confidentiality guidelines/standards of, 10, 24, 97n4; recommendations on destruction of patient records, 29; resource information from, 92–93, 94, 95
American Hospital Association (AHA), *Patient's Bill of Rights,* 9–10, 97n3
Answering machines, confidentiality risks with, 62–63
Attorneys, information policies and procedures for, 40
Authorization for release of health information, 37–39; dating of, 13, 37, 39, 98n9; revocation of, 39; sample, 38; signature on, 13, 37, 98n8; of substance

abuse patients, 12–14, 98nn8–9; waiver of, 46

## B

Brandt, M., 26, 36, 39

## C

Carpenter, J., 77
Case law, on confidentiality and privacy, 22–24
Cellular phones, confidentiality risks with, 63–64
Claims data, to determine extent of confidentiality problem, 31
Computer-Based Patient Record Institute (CPRI), 88, 91, 94
Computerized patient information: controlling access to, 5, 25–26, 27, 50–51, 77; difficulty of maintaining confidentiality of, 5–6; environment-related confidentiality risks with, 33, 52–53, 87; hardware-related confidentiality risks with, 33, 48–50, 84–86; human-related confidentiality risks with, 34, 53, 87–88; proposed federal standards for security of, 10, 15–20; on psychiatric treatment, 1, 97n1; software-related confidentiality risks with, 33, 50–52, 86–87. *See also* Health information; Medical records
Confidentiality: case law on, 22–24; federal laws and regulations on, 11–15; future of, of health information, 77–80;

Confidentiality, *continued*
operational difficulties in protecting, 4–6; organizational information requiring, 10–11; portion of health information requiring, 10, 36, 44, 98n10; professional standards on, 9–10, 24, 97nn2, 4; public concern about, 1–2; resources on, 79, 90–96; of substance abuse records, 12–14, 44, 98nn8–10. *See also* Privacy

Confidentiality breaches: common behaviors resulting in, 26–29; extent of, 7; implications of, 7–8; media reports on, 29–30; preventing, 32. *See also* Confidentiality risks; Risk assessment

Confidentiality risks: with e-mail and Internet access, 53–58; environment-related, 33, 52–53, 87; with facsimile (fax) machines, 59–61; hardware-related, 33, 48–50, 84–86; human-related, 34, 53, 87–88; methods of determining extent of, 30–31; with multimedia records, 64–65; organizational climate-related, 33, 67–69, 84; with pagers, 61; software-related, 33, 50–52, 86–87; with telemedicine, 61–62; with telephone and associated technologies, 62–64. *See also* Confidentiality breaches; Risk assessment

Confidentiality training, 67–76; for employees, 5, 69–72; hindrances to, 67–69; for physicians, 74–76; for vendors, 73–74; for volunteers, 72–73

Coroners, information policies and procedures for, 42

Courts, information policies and procedures for, 40–41

Curran, K., 27

Curran, M., 27

**D**

Data remanence, 49–50

Date, on authorizations for release of health information, 13, 37, 39, 98n9

Digital imaging, confidentiality risks with, 64–65

*Doe* v. *Methodist Hospital,* 23

Drug abuse records. *See* Substance abuse records

**E**

E-mail: confidentiality risks with, 53–55; sample guidelines on, 55–57

Electronic signatures, proposed standards on, 15–20

Electronically maintained health information. *See* Computerized patient information

Emergency Treatment and Labor Act, 43

Employee, surveys of, to determine extent of confidentiality problem, 30–31

Employees: access by, and confidentiality protection, 4–5; access to psychiatric records by, 1, 97n1; confidentiality training for, 5, 69–72; information policies and procedures for, 42–43; risk assessment involvement by, 81–84, 88–89

Employers, information policies and procedures for, 41

Encryption, 51

Environmental risks, assessing, 33, 52–53, 87

Equifax, 3, 7

*Estate of Behringer* v. *Princeton Medical Center,* 22

Ethical standards, on confidentiality of health information, 9–10

**F**

Facsimile (fax) machines: confidentiality risks with, 59–61; precautions when using, 59; resource on, 91

Family of patient: health information access by, 4; information policies and procedures for, 41–42

Federal laws and regulations, on confidentiality, 11–15

Federal privacy rule, proposed, 10, 20–22; on authorizations for release of information, 36, 38, 39; confidentiality and security training requirements of, 71;

on disclosing health information to various information users, 40–41, 42, 43, 44, 46; on patients' access to their health information, 45

Federal standards on security and electronic signatures, proposed, 10, 15–20; health information definition in, 11; steps in developing and implementing, 15

Freedom of Information Act (FOIA), 11–12

Funeral homes, information policies and procedures for, 42

## G

Givens, B., 2, 7

Government, federal: confidentiality laws and regulations of, 11–15; information policies and procedures for oversight agencies of, 42; proposed privacy rule of, 10, 20–22; proposed security and electronic signature standards of, 10, 15–20; response by, to public concern about privacy, 3–4

Grostick, S., 36

Guest relations data, to determine extent of confidentiality problem, 31

## H

Hanken, M. A., 36

Hardware-related risks, assessing, 33, 48–50, 84–86

Harris poll, on public's concern about privacy, 3, 7

Harvard Community Health Plan, accessibility of psychiatric records in, 1, 97n1

Health Care Financing Administration (HCFA): proposed definition of health information, 11; risk assessment mandated by, 32. See also Federal privacy rule, proposed; Federal standards on security and electronic signatures, proposed

Health Care Information Management Systems Society (HIMSS), 94

Health Care Personal Information Nondisclosure Act, 44, 98n12

Health care providers: confidentiality training for, 74–76; information policies and procedures for, 42–43

Health Care Reform Task Forces, 3

Health information: access to, 4–5, 26; consumer expectation of privacy of, 1–2; future of confidentiality of, 77–80; general principles on release of, 35–39; Health Care Financing Administration's definition of, 11; individually identifiable, proposed federal rule on privacy of, 10, 20–22; ownership of, 36; sold or used for commercial advantage, 78, 98n12; standards on confidentiality of, 9–10; types of users of, 39–47. See also Computerized patient information; Medical records

Health information releases/disclosures: general principles of, 35–39; "minimum necessary" standard for, 20–21, 43; "need to know" basis for, 43; to various types of information users, 39–47. See also Access

Health insurance companies, information policies and procedures for, 44

Health Insurance Portability and Accountability Act (HIPAA), 4, 14–15

Health maintenance organizations (HMOs), accessibility of psychiatric records in, 1, 97n1

Hippocratic oath, 9, 97n2

Human factor risks, assessing, 34, 53, 87–88

## I

Improvement committees: confidentiality of records of, 11; information policies and procedures for, 45–46

Incident reports: to determine extent of confidentiality problem, 31; as requiring confidentiality, 10–11

Indian Health Service facilities, 12

Information disasters, preventing, with risk assessments, 32

Information releases/disclosures. See Health information releases/disclosures

Information technology: confidentiality risks associated with various types of, 53–65; impact of, on confidentiality, 5–6. *See also* Computerized patient information

Information users, writing policies and procedures for various, 39–47

Integrated health care delivery systems, as impacting confidentiality, 6

International Computer Security Associations, 88

Internet: confidentiality risks with access to, 53–55; future of health information confidentiality and, 78; resources available on, 95–96; sample guidelines on using, 55–57

**J**

Jacobs, E., 36

Joint Commission on Accreditation of Healthcare Organizations (JCAHO), 9, 88, 93, 94

**K**

Kallail, K. J., 28

Kitson, J., 27

**L**

LaPorte Hospital (Indiana), 77

Law enforcement, information policies and procedures for, 40–41

Laws, federal, on confidentiality, 11–12, 14–15. *See also* Case law; Federal privacy rule, proposed

"Least privilege" principle for accessing health information, 26

Listservs, 54–55

**M**

Managed care, as impacting confidentiality, 6

McCann, R., 11

Media: attention given confidentiality in, 2; confidentiality breaches reported in, 29–30; information policies and procedures for, 44–45

Medical examiners, information policies and procedures for, 42

Medical Information Bureau (MIB), 2, 3

Medical Information Privacy and Security Act, 44

Medical records: confidential, destruction/disposal of, 28–29; confidential vs. nonconfidential information in, 10, 36, 44, 98n10; psychiatric, 1, 7, 97n1; substance abuse, 10, 12–14, 44, 98nn8–10. *See also* Computerized patient information; Health information

*Methodist Hospital, Doe* v., 23

"Minimum necessary" standard for information disclosure, 20–21, 43

Monetary losses, preventing, with risk assessments, 33

Multimedia records, confidentiality risks with, 64–65

**N**

National Computer Security Association, 59–60

"Need to know" basis for information disclosure, 43

News media. *See* Media

**O**

Occurrence reports. *See* Incident reports

*O'Connor* v. *Rutland Medical Center,* 23

Organizational climate: as hindrance to confidentiality, 67–69; risk assessment of, 33, 84

Organizational information, requiring confidentiality, 10–11

Organizations: confidentiality and privacy standards of, 9–10, 97nn3–4; resource, 94–95

**P**

Pagers, confidentiality risks with, 61

Password problems, 51

Patient ombudsman program data, to determine extent of confidentiality problem, 31

Patient records. *See* Medical records

Patient satisfaction surveys, to determine extent of confidentiality problem, 31
Patients, information policies and procedures for, 45
Photographs, confidentiality risks with, 64–65
Physicians: confidentiality training for, 74–76; information policies and procedures for, 42–43
Portable phones, confidentiality risks with, 63–64
Press, Ganey Associates, 31
*Princeton Medical Center, Estate of Behringer v.*, 22
Privacy: American Hospital Association's *Patient's Bill of Rights* on, 9–10, 97n3; case law on, 22–24; consumer expectations of, of health information, 1–2; proposed federal rule on, of individually identifiable health information, 10, 20–22; public concern about, 3; resources on, 90–96. *See also* Confidentiality
Privacy Act of 1974, 12
Privacy Rights Clearinghouse, 94–95
Psychiatric records. *See* Medical records
Public health departments, information policies and procedures for, 42
Public image problems, preventing, with risk assessments, 32

**Q**

Quality review committees: confidentiality of records of, 11; information policies and procedures for, 45–46

**R**

Rankin, B., 23, 24
Regulations, federal, on confidentiality of substance abuse records, 12–14, 98nn8–9
Researchers, information policies and procedures for, 46–47
Resources, 90–96; associations and organizations, 94–95; printed materials, 91–93; software, 94; videotapes, 93–94

Risk assessment, 81–90; areas of risk examined in, 33–34, 48–53, 84–88; benefits of, 90; mandated by Health Care Financing Administration, 32; need for repeating, 90; reasons for doing, 31–33; resources on conducting, 88; staff involvement in, 81–84, 88–89; using results of, 89–90. *See also* Confidentiality breaches; Confidentiality risks
*Rutland Medical Center, O'Connor v.*, 23

**S**

*St. Clare's Hospital, Velasquez v.*, 23
Security, proposed federal rule on, of electronically maintained health information, 10, 15–20
Signatures: on authorizations for disclosure of substance abuse records, 13, 98n8; on authorizations for release of health information, 37; electronic, proposed rule on, 10, 15–20
Social Security Act, Administrative Simplification amendment to, 14–15
Software-related risks, assessing, 33, 50–52, 86–87
Students, information policies and procedures for, 47
Substance abuse records: confidential portion of, 10, 44, 98n10; regulations on confidentiality of, 12–14, 98nn8–9

**T**

Task Force on Privacy, 3
Taylor, D. K., 27
Technology. *See* Information technology
Telemedicine, confidentiality risks with, 61–62
Telephone and associated technologies, confidentiality risks with, 62–64
Training. *See* Confidentiality training

**U**

Ullom-Minnich, P. D., 28
U.S. Department of Defense health care facilities, 12

U.S. Department of Health and Human Services (USDHHS), 4, 6; proposed privacy and security standards from, 15–22; Task Force on Privacy, 3; Workgroup on Electronic Data Interchange (WEDI), 3

## V

Velasquez, N., 7
*Velasquez* v. *St. Clare's Hospital,* 23
Vendors, confidentiality training for, 73–74
Veterans' Administration health facilities, 12

Videotapes: confidentiality risks with, 64–65; as resources, 93–94
Viruses, computer, 51–52
Voice mail, confidentiality risks with, 62–63
Volunteers, confidentiality training for, 72–73

## W

Waiver of authorization, 46
Websites, offering confidentiality information, 79, 95–96
Workgroup on Electronic Data Interchange (WEDI), 3